FROM BEDSIDE TO BOARDROOM:
A GUIDE TO NURSING LEADERSHIP

Quaternary Healthcare Consultancy, LLC

COPYRIGHT © 2025

DISCLAIMER

Disclaimer Notice: Please note the information contained within this document is for educational and entertainment purposes only. All effort has been executed to present accurate, up to date, reliable, complete information. No warranties of any kind are declared or implied. Readers acknowledge that the author is not engaged in the rendering of legal, financial, medical or professional advice.

The content within this book has been derived from various sources. Please consult a licensed professional before attempting any techniques outlined in this book. By reading this document, the reader agrees that under no circumstances is the author responsible for any losses, direct or indirect, that are incurred as a result of the use of the information contained within this document, including, but not limited to, errors, omissions, or inaccuracies.

https://www.quaternaryconsultant.com

Acknowledgment

This book is a testament to the incredible mentors who shaped my journey, and I owe a profound debt of gratitude to three extraordinary nurses—Paula, Lori, and Jean.

Paula, thank you for having confidence to hire me into my first Perioperative job. Your patience and expertise laid the foundation for my perioperative career.

Lori, you taught me not just the technical skills, but the deeper understanding of what it means to be a nurse in the OR—focused, compassionate, and always prepared.

Jean, your steady guidance and scrub expertise made all the difference.

Furthermore, my career was shaped and honed by the unwavering support, encouragement, and inspiration of three incredible colleagues and lifelong friends: Monica, Christy, and Erik.

Finally, a huge thank you to my family and friends, especially my husband Dr. Richard Kidd.

Because of all of you, I not only became a perioperative nurse, but I found my calling in leadership, transformation, and mentorship. Your influence continues to shape the work I do today, and I am forever grateful.

TABLE OF CONTENT

INTRODUCTION

Leadership in nursing is not a role many set out to achieve when they begin their careers. For most nursing professionals, the initial focus is on patient care—those vital, immediate moments that define the essence of the profession. Yet, as time passes, nurses often find themselves drawn into roles that require more than clinical expertise and much more than bedside manners. They are asked to manage teams, implement policies, and make decisions that impact not only individual patients but entire units and sometimes, entire organizations.

This natural evolution can present itself as both a challenge and an opportunity. It's no secret that healthcare systems around the world are at a crossroads. Recent shortages in staffing, the rapid advancement of medical technologies, and growing patient populations demand leaders who can navigate these complexities with confidence and foresight. For nurses, this means stepping out of their comfort zones and into a world where their voices and decisions carry weight far beyond the bedside.

Consider this: how often are the best bedside nurses unexpectedly tapped for leadership roles without formal preparation? It's a scenario many in the profession can relate to. While every nurse leader's journey is unique, many share a common starting point: an unforeseen opportunity. For me, the path to leadership began with a simple request. Like many nurse managers, I found that excelling at my job meant being entrusted with special projects and additional responsibilities. One day, my director called me into the office and asked if I would step in as the "interim" manager until a replacement could be found. Five years later, I was still the manager.

This story resonates because it reflects a fundamental truth in nursing: the transition into leadership is often unplanned, and the resources to succeed are rarely handed to you. While ambition and drive are vital, leadership cannot be rushed, particularly in healthcare. Millennials and Gen Z nurses often value purpose, flexibility, and innovation—qualities that make them uniquely suited for leadership. However, these generations sometimes desire to step into leadership roles immediately after college. The reality is that leadership isn't just about holding a title; it requires a deep understanding of the complexities of patient care, team dynamics, and organizational systems—knowledge best gained through hands-on, on-the-job experience.

Having solid clinical expertise and practical experience in your specialty is essential before transitioning into leadership. Not only does this prepare you for the challenges ahead, but it also builds credibility with your team. Nurses respect leaders who've walked in their shoes, made tough clinical decisions, and know the realities of the profession. Leadership isn't about skipping steps; it's about climbing the ladder with purpose, ensuring you have the tools and experience needed to support those you lead.

What makes this reality even more pressing is the impact of leadership—or the lack thereof—on patient outcomes and workplace culture. Strong leaders inspire teams, foster collaboration, and drive innovation. They act as the bridge between staff and administration, ensuring that policies make sense on the ground and that the voices of nurses are heard in decision-making rooms. Conversely, a gap in leadership can lead to burnout, high turnover, and strained patient care.

So, you may be wondering why you picked up this book, or why your friend, family member, or coworker gave it to you. You're asking yourself, Why does this book matter? Well, this book was written to address these challenges head-on. It's not just a guide—it's a call to action. Leadership in nursing has the power to transform healthcare systems, but only if leaders are equipped with the tools and knowledge to succeed.

The journey from bedside to leadership is often marked by uncertainty, with little formal guidance to ease the transition.

While nursing education provides a foundation in theory, the practical realities of leading a team, managing resources, and influencing change are skills that often must be learned on the job.

For nurses stepping into leadership roles, the stakes are high. Patient safety, team morale, and organizational efficiency often rest on their shoulders. Yet many nurses feel unprepared for these responsibilities, unsure of how to navigate the complexities of healthcare leadership. This book bridges that gap, offering actionable strategies and real-world insights to empower aspiring leaders to thrive.

As healthcare evolves, it's clear that different generations approach leadership with unique perspectives. Generally, Millennials often see leadership as a way to make a meaningful impact while creating stability in their careers. They value transparency, collaboration, and inclusivity, all of which are essential in modern nursing leadership. Stepping into leadership allows them to tackle systemic inefficiencies, advocate for their teams, and foster supportive workplace cultures.

For most Gen Z nurses, the draw to leadership generally lies in innovation and purpose. Digital natives with a natural inclination toward technology, they see the potential for telemedicine, data analytics, and other tools to revolutionize healthcare. They are the most likely to challenge traditional methods, advocating for bold, forward-thinking approaches to leadership. By embracing flexibility and cultivating a culture where change is welcomed, they bring a dynamic energy to nursing leadership that has the potential to drive real transformation.

By recognizing these generational differences, this book offers strategies that resonate with both groups. Whether you're a Millennial striving to build a supportive team culture, a Gen Z nurse eager to disrupt outdated systems, or a nursing professional that falls between the lines, the insights here will help you embrace leadership in a way that aligns with your values and aspirations.

Leadership is more than just a professional milestone—it's a journey of personal growth, self-discovery, and transformation. For nurses, this journey often begins with a single step, whether it's taking on additional responsibilities, guiding a colleague through a tough situation, or realizing that your voice has the power to influence change. Leadership isn't about titles; it's about the impact you have on others and the vision you bring to the table.

Yet the journey to leadership isn't without its difficulties. Transitioning from bedside care to a leadership role means stepping into uncharted territory. Suddenly, you're not just responsible for your own work but for the performance and well-being of your entire team. You're tasked with making decisions that ripple through the organization, balancing the demands of patients, staff, and administration. It's a role that requires resilience, adaptability, and a commitment to continuous learning.

For many nurses, leadership begins with a moment of doubt. You ask yourself: Am I ready for this? Can I really lead others? These questions are natural, but they are also the first step on a transformative journey—one that will not only shape your career but also enrich your understanding of yourself and your ability to impact others. Leadership in nursing isn't just about managing tasks; it's about becoming a force for positive change.

The transition from bedside care to leadership is a leap of faith. It's stepping into a role where you are no longer focused solely on individual patients but on the well-being of an entire team—and, by extension, every patient they touch. It's about looking beyond the immediate challenges and envisioning solutions that benefit the whole organization.

Each decision you make as a leader has the potential to shape not only your team's performance but also the culture of your workplace. Great leaders inspire those around them, creating environments where collaboration thrives and where every team member feels empowered to contribute their best.

The Growth Leadership Brings

One of the most rewarding aspects of this journey is the opportunity for personal growth. Leadership challenges you to develop skills you may not have thought you needed: resilience, strategic thinking, and the ability to see challenges as opportunities. It encourages self-reflection and helps you uncover strengths you didn't realize you had. Along the way, you'll also learn from your missteps—each one a lesson that shapes the kind of leader you want to become.

Of course, the journey isn't always easy. The weight of responsibility can feel heavy, and the learning curve can be steep. But with each challenge, you'll find yourself becoming more confident, more adaptable, and more capable. As you guide your team through obstacles and celebrate their successes, you'll come to see leadership not just as a role but as a calling.

Leadership also offers a unique opportunity to leave a lasting impact. As a nurse leader, you have the power to shape the careers of those you mentor, the policies you advocate for, and the standards of care you uphold. Your influence extends far beyond the immediate tasks of the day, rippling through the organization and even the profession as a whole.

This is particularly important for today's nurses. For example, Millennials, who often seek to create supportive and inclusive workplaces, can use leadership to build environments where their teams feel valued and empowered. Gen Z nurses, with their passion for innovation, see leadership as a platform to challenge outdated systems and drive change. Together, these generations are redefining what it means to lead in healthcare, making it not just a responsibility but an opportunity to transform the field.

Now, I know I've said it before, but Millennials and Gen Z really are changing the game. Millennials are all about creating communities where everyone feels they belong, and Gen Z? They're out here tearing down old systems and asking, "But why do we do it this way?" Honestly, they're not just stepping into leadership—they're shaking it up, and it's exciting to see where they'll take us.

A Roadmap to Leadership

Leadership is like trying to assemble furniture from a certain popular Swedish store—you start with enthusiasm, but soon you're staring at an instruction manual that's more confusing than helpful, wondering why you ever thought this was a good idea. Thankfully, this book is designed to be a little less frustrating than assembling a bookshelf. It's here to guide you step by step, helping you build the confidence, skills, and vision needed to succeed as a leader in nursing.

As you step into this role, remember that leadership is as much about the journey as it is about the destination. It's a process of continuous learning and growth, of embracing challenges and celebrating victories. Whether you're just beginning to explore your leadership potential or already taking your first steps in a new role, this book will guide you with actionable strategies, relatable stories, and the tools you need to succeed.

The journey may be demanding, but it's also one of the most fulfilling paths you can take. Leadership isn't about being perfect; it's about striving to be better every day—for yourself, your team, and your patients. The rewards of this journey go far beyond professional accomplishments; they lie in the lives you touch and the legacy you leave behind.

The Promise of What Lies Ahead

This journey isn't about perfection. Let's face it—no leader gets it right every time. It's about learning, growing, and figuring out how to use what you have to make a difference. Leadership is messy, rewarding, challenging, and transformative all at once. The chapters ahead will help you navigate the ups and downs, offering tools and strategies that empower you to lead with purpose, even on the days when everything feels like it's falling apart.

This book isn't just about teaching you the "how" of leadership. It's about helping you discover your unique strengths and approach to leading others. You'll learn to build trust, foster collaboration, and create a work environment that not only supports your team but also inspires them to grow.

You'll also learn how to navigate change—a constant in healthcare. From staffing shortages to implementing new technologies, nurse leaders are at the forefront of managing transitions. With the right tools and mindset, you'll be prepared to guide your team through these challenges with confidence and resilience.

What You'll Find in This Book

Think of this book as your roadmap. Leadership may feel like a winding path filled with unexpected detours, but with the right guide, you'll navigate it with confidence. Here's a glimpse of what lies ahead:

- **Discovering Your Leadership Potential:** It all begins with recognizing that you have what it takes to lead. You'll explore the qualities that make great leaders and identify your own strengths and areas for growth. Don't worry—there's no judgment here, just a supportive push to get you started.

•**Building Essential Skills:** Leadership isn't just about big-picture thinking. It's about mastering the nuts and bolts that make a team run smoothly. You'll learn how to communicate effectively (even with that one coworker who seems to speak in riddles), manage your time like a pro, and make decisions that inspire trust.

•**Navigating Challenges and Change:** Let's be real—healthcare is a constantly shifting landscape. Policies change, technologies evolve, and sometimes it feels like you're juggling flaming swords. This book will teach you how to adapt, stay calm under pressure, and lead your team through tough times with resilience and grace.

•**Inspiring Your Team:** Leadership isn't about barking orders from a mountaintop. It's about creating an environment where your team feels valued, supported, and motivated. You'll learn how to build trust, foster collaboration, and celebrate the unique strengths each person brings to the table.

•**Advocating for Change:** As a nurse leader, you're in a powerful position to influence policy, improve workplace culture, and drive innovations that benefit both patients and staff. You'll discover how to use your voice effectively, ensuring that the needs of your team and your profession are heard.

•**Creating Your Leadership Legacy:** Leadership isn't just about what you achieve today—it's about the impact you leave behind. This book will help you define your vision, set meaningful goals, and build a legacy that inspires future generations of nurses.

Why Leadership Matters More Than Ever

The world of healthcare is changing rapidly, and leadership has never been more important. Every decision a nurse leader makes—whether it's implementing a new workflow or supporting a struggling team member—has a ripple effect that can shape patient outcomes, workplace culture, and even the broader healthcare system.

The stakes are high, but the rewards are immense. Nurse leaders have the opportunity to create environments where staff feel supported, patients receive exceptional care, and innovation thrives. It's a chance to make a tangible difference, not just for today but for years to come.

But let's not sugarcoat it—leadership can also be exhausting. Some days, it might feel like you're trying to herd cats while simultaneously putting out fires (literal or metaphorical). On those days, it's important to remember why you started this journey in the first place. Leadership is about more than just keeping things running; it's about inspiring others, solving problems, and leaving the world of healthcare better than you found it.

This book isn't going to pretend that leadership is all sunshine and rainbows. There will be moments when you question your sanity, your career choices, and possibly even your favorite coffee order. That's okay—it's part of the process. You're not alone in those moments of doubt, and this book is here to remind you that every leader, even the ones who seem like they have it all figured out, started where you are now.

Leadership also comes with its fair share of unexpected surprises. For example, you might find yourself becoming an expert in deciphering cryptic emails or navigating office politics. You'll probably learn more about budgeting than you ever wanted to know, and you'll definitely develop a new appreciation for the phrase "other duties as assigned." But through it all, you'll also discover strengths you didn't know you had and build relationships that make the challenges worth it.

How This Book Will Support You

Leadership in nursing often feels like being handed a map without directions. One moment you're excelling at bedside care, and the next, you're supposed to lead meetings, manage teams, and fix problems you didn't create—all while keeping your sanity intact. Here's what you can expect:

Practical Strategies: Let's face it—no one becomes a great leader by winging it. Leadership requires skills that aren't always second nature, like managing conflict without flipping a table, delegating tasks without micromanaging, and balancing the competing demands of patient care and team morale. This book is packed with strategies that work in real life, not just in theory. Whether it's surviving a tough meeting or coaching a struggling team member, you'll find solutions you can apply immediately. Think of these as your "nurse manager survival tools"—because duct tape isn't always an option.

Relatable Stories: Ever feel like you're the only one who doesn't have it all figured out? Spoiler alert: You're not. This book features stories from real nurse leaders who've faced the same challenges you're tackling. You'll read about missteps, triumphs, and everything in between—like the time someone accidentally called a team huddle in the supply closet because they forgot where the conference room was. These stories remind you that you're not alone, and more importantly, that success isn't about getting it right the first time. It's about learning, adapting, and showing up again tomorrow.

Reflection Exercises: If you've ever looked in the mirror and wondered, Am I really cut out for this? —good news, you're not alone. Leadership isn't about knowing all the answers; it's about being willing to ask the right questions, starting with yourself. Each chapter includes reflection exercises designed to help you dig deep, discover your strengths, and confront the areas where growth is needed. Don't worry, no one's grading you—this is for your eyes only (and maybe a coffee-stained notebook). These prompts are like a pep talk from your future self, reminding you why you're in this role and how far you've come.

Inspiration: Let's be real: leadership can feel like herding cats, and some days it's tempting to just throw in the towel and find a quiet corner to cry in. That's why this book is infused with moments of inspiration—quotes from great leaders, insights that reframe your perspective, and reminders that even on your worst day, you're making a difference. These are the breadcrumbs of motivation that will help you keep going, even when the coffee machine breaks, the Wi-Fi crashes, and someone just asks you to fix something that clearly requires an IT degree.

At its core, this book isn't about making you a flawless leader—it's about helping you grow into a more intentional one. Whether you're mentoring a new nurse, leading a brainstorming session, or advocating for much-needed change, this book will equip you with the tools and confidence to lead with purpose and heart.

Looking Ahead

Leadership is more of a scenic hike than a sprint. There will be detours, uphill climbs, and moments when you question why you even started. But along the way, you'll also discover breathtaking views—like the time your team pulled together to solve a crisis or when a struggling nurse you mentored finally finds their stride. These victories remind you that the climb is worth it.

This journey isn't just about solving problems or meeting goals; it's about becoming the kind of leader others look up to. And if that sounds intimidating, don't worry—you don't have to do it alone. This book will be your guide, offering advice, encouragement, and the occasional laugh when you need it most. Leadership might be serious business, but it doesn't have to be boring.

As you turn the page, remember this: Leadership isn't about where you start—it's about where you're willing to go. You've already taken the first step by picking up this book, which shows your willingness to grow and lead with intention. That's a big deal—and one worth celebrating.

So, here's to the adventure ahead. Let's embrace the challenges, learn from the missteps, and celebrate the wins (yes, even the small ones). Together, we'll navigate this unpredictable, rewarding journey called leadership—and who knows? Maybe we'll even have some fun along the way.

Now, let's get started by exploring the foundational qualities that define great leaders and uncovering practical ways to recognize and nurture your own leadership potential!

PART 1

BUILDING THE FOUNDATION FOR LEADERSHIP

CHAPTER 1

RECOGNIZING LEADERSHIP POTENTIAL

Early in my career, I worked with a nurse named Carla who was initially very shy and reserved. When she first joined our team, she rarely spoke up during rounds, and it was clear she felt unsure of herself in high-pressure situations. She preferred to observe, quietly absorbing the dynamics of the unit, rather than actively participating. It would have been easy to overlook her; to assume she wasn't leadership material. But something remarkable happened over time. Carla took ownership of her personal growth—she enrolled in communication workshops, actively sought feedback from senior staff, and found a mentor who believed in her potential, even when she doubted it herself.

This self-directed growth wasn't just about acquiring new skills; it was about cultivating a leadership mindset. She began to see challenges not as obstacles, but as opportunities for learning and development. This shift in perspective was crucial.

One day, during a particularly chaotic emergency situation, our charge nurse was unexpectedly called away, leaving the team in disarray. The usual hierarchy dissolved into confusion. It was in this moment of crisis that Carla, despite being one of the quieter nurses on the team, calmly stepped forward. She didn't shout orders or try to take complete control; instead, she assessed the situation, organized the staff, and ensured that patient needs were prioritized. She became the calm in the storm. It was a turning point, not only in that specific situation but also in Carla's leadership journey. From that day forward, she became one of the most dependable and respected leaders on our floor.

Carla's story is a powerful reminder that leadership isn't about being the loudest voice in the room or having decades of experience. It's not about charisma or extroversion. It's about developing key qualities, recognizing opportunities to contribute, and being willing to take action when it counts. It's about recognizing the potential within oneself and in others, even when it's hidden beneath a quiet exterior.

Understanding Leadership Qualities in Nursing

Leadership in nursing is not about the title you hold or the position you're given. It's about the influence you have, the way you guide your team, and how you advocate for your patients. As Carla's experience illustrates, effective leadership in nursing is rooted in a few key qualities that transcend rank, experience, and personality.

These core qualities—communication, empathy, and resilience—are essential for fostering trust, creating collaborative environments, and maintaining quality patient care. But perhaps even more fundamental is the capacity for self-awareness and a commitment to continuous growth.

Communication

One of the most vital aspects of leadership is communication. Effective leaders understand that their role isn't just about giving orders but about ensuring their team is well-informed, heard, and aligned in their goals. Whether you're explaining a treatment plan to a patient, giving instructions to a nursing team, or managing conflict between staff, how you communicate can make or break the situation. Clear, open, and honest communication helps prevent errors, build trust, and enhance team morale.

Consider a nurse leader who always makes it a priority to clearly explain new procedures to their team, answering questions and providing clarification. Their approach reduces confusion and helps the team perform their duties more effectively. This is what good communication can do—it facilitates collaboration, reduces mistakes, and inspires confidence.

Empathy

Leadership is not only about making decisions but about understanding the impact those decisions have on others. Empathy is a cornerstone of emotional intelligence, and it's crucial in nursing. Empathetic leaders know how to relate to others on a deeper level. They recognize that behind every clinical task is a person with individual needs, struggles, and goals.

Take for instance a nurse manager who notices one of their team members is looking stressed. Instead of pushing them harder, they take a moment to check in, offering support or even adjusting their workload temporarily. This small act of empathy boosts team morale and encourages loyalty. When leaders show empathy, they create environments where people feel understood, respected, and supported.

Resilience

This can be described as the ability to recover from setbacks, adapt to changes, and keep moving forward, even in the face of adversity. Nursing is a demanding field, and the challenges can be overwhelming. A resilient leader doesn't buckle under pressure—they rise to the occasion. They remain calm and steady, which helps their team do the same. In times of crisis or stress, it's the resilient leader who sets the tone, models a positive attitude, and helps the team navigate challenges with strength.

A Story on The Power of Empathy and Resilience

A nurse leader, Sarah, was known for her remarkable ability to remain calm and supportive, even in the most intense moments. During one particularly challenging night shift, the unit was hit with an overwhelming number of patients. Staff were stretched thin, and the pressure was palpable.

Sarah walked into the chaos, her calm demeanor cutting through the tension. Instead of dictating orders, she took the time to check in with each nurse, ensuring they felt supported. One nurse, in particular, appeared visibly exhausted, and Sarah pulled her aside for a brief conversation. Rather than simply asking how she was doing, Sarah listened—really listened. Together, they made a plan to shift some tasks and gave the nurse a moment to collect herself. This simple act of empathy alleviated stress for the nurse and created a ripple effect of calm throughout the team.

Later, when a difficult situation arose, Sarah's resilience became evident. Despite the mounting stress, she remained focused on the bigger picture—ensuring that both patient care and staff well-being were prioritized. By the end of the shift, the team was exhausted but grateful. They had followed Sarah's example, working together to get through the night. Her leadership wasn't about having all the answers—it was about providing the emotional and strategic support needed to keep the team grounded.

Building These Qualities

The good news is that these leadership qualities aren't innate—they can be developed over time. Here's how you can cultivate these skills:

Improving Communication Skills

Practice active listening: Give your full attention when someone speaks, and ask follow-up questions to show engagement.

***Be clear and concise*:** Whether writing emails or speaking with colleagues, make sure your message is direct and easy to understand.

***Give and receive feedback*:** Constructive feedback is key to growth, both for you and your team.

Cultivating Empathy

***Take the time to connect with others*:** Whether it's your patients or colleagues, listen to their concerns and validate their feelings.

***Step into others' shoes*:** Try to view situations from their perspective before responding.

***Offer emotional support*:** Check in with your team during stressful times and offer words of encouragement when needed.

Building Resilience:

Practice stress management techniques: Take regular breaks, practice deep breathing, or engage in mindfulness.

Learn from challenges: Instead of seeing setbacks as failures, use them as opportunities for growth.

Stay positive: Focus on what can be done rather than what can't.

In nursing leadership, communication, empathy, and resilience are the bedrock qualities that create strong leaders and strong teams. While they may not come naturally to everyone, they can be cultivated through intentional practice and commitment to growth. As a nurse, developing these qualities will not only help you step into leadership roles but also allow you to make a lasting, positive impact on your team and your patients.

*Busting Common Myths About Leadership in Nursing

It won't be a good guide, if we didn't venture into Myth-busting! Nursing Leadership is shrouded in misconceptions that can discourage talented individuals from stepping up. Many nurses believe that leadership is only for those in formal management roles, that it requires a specific personality type, or that leadership is something you're either born with or you're not. These myths can create barriers to leadership development and prevent nurses from realizing their own potential. In reality, leadership in nursing is a skill that anyone can develop, regardless of experience level, personality, or job title.

1. "Leadership is only for those in management positions."

It's easy to think that leadership is reserved for those with titles like "Nurse Manager" or "Charge Nurse." However, leadership happens at all levels in nursing. True leadership isn't about holding a formal title; it's about the impact you make on your team and your patients. Nurses who lead from the bedside—advocating for their patients, mentoring colleagues, and initiating positive changes in their units—are some of the most effective leaders. Whether you're in a management position or not, leadership is about influence, not authority.

For instance, a nurse working on a busy surgical unit might not have a "leader" title, but by mentoring new nurses, organizing team huddles, and facilitating communication among staff, they exhibit leadership every day. Their influence drives better teamwork and improves patient care, showing that leadership doesn't require a title—it requires action.

2. "You need to be an extrovert to be a great leader."

Many nurses assume that leaders need to be outgoing, gregarious, and naturally charismatic. However, introverts often make exceptional leaders due to their deep listening skills, thoughtful decision-making, and ability to connect with others on a one-on-one basis. Leadership is about understanding your team, making informed decisions, and fostering collaboration—qualities that introverts tend to excel at.

Take a nurse leader who is more reserved but is known for their ability to listen attentively and think critically under pressure. By considering all perspectives and making well-thought-out decisions, this leader creates an inclusive environment where everyone's voice is heard and respected. Introverted leaders build strong relationships, earning the respect and trust of their team in a quieter, but equally effective, way.

3. "Leaders are born, not made."

This myth suggests that you either have leadership qualities or you don't. In reality, leadership is a skill that can be developed over time. It's about learning, adapting, and growing. While some people may have natural leadership inclinations, anyone can cultivate the skills necessary for effective leadership through self-reflection, mentorship, and experience. Leadership isn't about being perfect—it's about being open to learning and improving.

4. "Leadership is all about telling people what to do."

There's a common misconception that leadership is about giving orders and exerting control. In fact, great leadership is about influence, collaboration, and inspiring others. Nurse leaders guide their teams by setting a positive example, empowering their colleagues, and encouraging collaboration. Rather than telling others what to do, effective leaders create an environment where everyone is motivated to contribute to the team's success.

5. "Only experienced nurses can be leaders."

It's easy to believe that leadership is something only experienced nurses can undertake. However, leadership potential exists in nurses at every stage of their career. Leadership isn't about how long you've been in the field; it's about how you approach your work and how you support others. Even new nurses can demonstrate leadership by taking initiative, seeking opportunities to improve patient care, and offering support to their peers.

6. "Leadership is a solo journey."

Finally, many people think that leadership is an individual endeavor—something you have to do alone. But in nursing, leadership is a team effort. Effective nurse leaders know that they don't have all the answers and seek support from their peers, mentors, and colleagues. Leadership is about collaboration, and the best leaders recognize the importance of teamwork, mentorship, and shared responsibility.

A nurse leader might frequently seek advice from more experienced colleagues, work closely with team members to solve problems, and encourage a supportive environment where everyone feels valued. By fostering a culture of collaboration and mentorship, they build stronger teams and improve patient outcomes.

In reality, research continues to challenge these myths about leadership in nursing. According to the *Journal of Nursing Management*, informal nurse leaders (those who may not hold formal leadership titles) have been shown to significantly impact workplace culture and patient outcomes. In fact, a study conducted by the *Nursing Times* found that 74% of nurses believe leadership development should begin at the bedside, not in management offices, reinforcing the idea that leadership is accessible to all nurses, regardless of title.

In addition, a study published by the *American Nurses Association (ANA)* shows that diverse leadership styles (including those of introverts and those early in their careers) contribute to more effective healthcare teams. The research supports the fact that leadership potential exists in every nurse—regardless of experience, personality, or job title.

The myths surrounding leadership in nursing are just that—myths. Leadership is for everyone, no matter your personality type, experience level, or formal title. By breaking down these misconceptions, we can open the door to leadership development for all nurses. Leadership isn't about being born a leader; it's about embracing the qualities and mindset that allow you to influence, inspire, and elevate those around you.

***Self-Assessment: Do You Have What It Takes?**

Becoming a leader in nursing doesn't happen overnight, and it doesn't depend solely on title or years of experience. Instead, it's about assessing your own qualities, recognizing areas for improvement, and making a commitment to growth. Self-assessment is the first step in identifying whether you're ready to take on leadership roles and, if not, how you can work toward becoming the kind of leader you want to be.

To understand your leadership potential, it's important to consider the core qualities that great nurse leaders embody, as discussed earlier. These qualities are often developed over time, but you can start assessing where you are today and what areas to focus on.

Leadership Self-Assessment Checklist

Rate yourself on a scale of 1 (Needs Improvement) to 5 (Excellent) for each statement below:

I communicate clearly and confidently in a variety of situations. (1 2 3 4 5)

I actively listen to my colleagues and respond with empathy. (1 2 3 4 5)

I remain calm and adaptable under pressure. (1 2 3 4 5)

I take initiative and seek opportunities to solve problems. (1 2 3 4 5)

I support and encourage my colleagues in their professional growth. (1 2 3 4 5)

I take responsibility for my actions and decisions. (1 2 3 4 5)

I can provide constructive feedback without hesitation. (1 2 3 4 5)

I embrace change and seek out opportunities to learn. (1 2 3 4 5)

I advocate for my patients and colleagues when needed. (1 2 3 4 5)

I set a positive example for others through my work ethic and attitude. (1 2 3 4 5)

Now that you've completed your self-assessment, take a moment to reflect on your scores and your responses to the questions. If you found yourself scoring higher in areas like communication and empathy, congratulations—you likely have strong leadership potential in those areas! However, if you found certain aspects challenging, don't worry—leadership is a skill that can always be developed and refined.

Remember, leadership isn't about perfection. It's about making consistent progress. If you noticed areas where you'd like to improve, consider setting specific, measurable goals to focus on those qualities. For example, if you feel you could work on decision-making under pressure, you might set a goal to practice making quicker decisions in low-risk scenarios or seek guidance from mentors on how they navigate decision-making.

Practical Tips for Growth:

Seek Mentorship: Find a nurse leader you admire and ask them for guidance. Learn from their experiences and insights to improve your own leadership skills.

Take on Small Leadership Roles: Look for opportunities to lead within your current role, whether it's leading a team meeting, organizing a shift, or mentoring a new nurse.

Stay Open to Feedback: Be open to receiving feedback from your colleagues and supervisors. Constructive criticism can be incredibly valuable in your growth journey.

Invest in Continuous Learning: Attend leadership workshops, read books on leadership development, or join leadership-focused groups or committees to sharpen your skills.

> ***Florence Nightingale*** *– "I attribute my success to this—I never gave or took any excuse."*

Developing Leadership Skills in Everyday Practice

Leadership in nursing isn't just about managing teams or making high-level decisions; it's about how you approach each task, interaction, and challenge in your everyday work. Nightingale recognized the importance of responsibility and accountability in leadership. She didn't make excuses for her circumstances; she took initiative and led by example.

Whether you're organizing patient care, supporting colleagues, or responding to emergencies, leadership can be practiced and honed in the smallest moments. The beauty of nursing leadership is that it's not confined to boardrooms or management meetings—it's something you can demonstrate every day, often in the most unexpected ways.

1. Leading by Example

One of the most powerful ways to develop leadership skills is to simply **lead by example**. Every day, you have the opportunity to demonstrate qualities like integrity, accountability, empathy, and professionalism—qualities that are essential for any leader. When you model the behavior you expect from others, you set a standard for your team and create a culture of respect and accountability.

Practical Tips:

Set a high standard for yourself: Whether it's your work ethic, your attitude toward challenges, or your communication style, make sure you're holding yourself to the standard you want to see in others.

Stay calm under pressure: Nursing can be chaotic, but your ability to remain composed in difficult situations will inspire your team to do the same.

Model professionalism: Always maintain professionalism, no matter the circumstances. Your conduct sets the tone for your colleagues and your patients.

2. Inspiring Others Through Action

Leadership is about inspiring others to take action. As a nurse, you likely find yourself in situations where your team members are looking to you for guidance or reassurance. How you respond to these moments can have a significant impact on those around you. **Inspiring leadership** isn't about giving orders—it's about motivating others to step up, trust in their abilities, and perform their best.

Practical Tips:

Encourage your colleagues: Take the time to praise your peers for their efforts, whether big or small. Recognition and appreciation can go a long way in motivating others.

Empower others to lead: Encourage your colleagues to take on leadership roles, even in small ways. Empowering others to step up not only builds their confidence but strengthens the entire team.

Foster a sense of teamwork: Promote collaboration and support, particularly during challenging moments. Strong teams are built on trust and shared responsibility.

3. Mentorship: Learning and Growing Together

Another key way to develop leadership skills is through **mentorship**—both as a mentor and as a mentee. Once again, I may sound like a broken record, but mentorship is really where it's at. Even if you're not yet in an official leadership role, mentorship can be a great opportunity to practice guiding others while also continuing your own growth.

Being a mentor means sharing your knowledge and experience with others, offering advice, and supporting them as they develop their skills. On the flip side, being a mentee allows you to learn from those with more experience, gain valuable insights, and refine your own leadership style. Mentorship is a two-way street—it helps you grow just as much as it helps the person you're guiding.

As you mentor others, you also learn the importance of listening, offering constructive feedback, and adapting your approach to meet the needs of different people. This helps you develop the flexibility and emotional intelligence that are critical for strong leadership.

Practical Tips:

Seek mentorship: Look for someone you respect and admire within your organization, and ask them to be your mentor. Take advantage of their experience and insights to help guide your development.

Be a mentor to others: Even if you don't hold a formal leadership role, you can still mentor new nurses or those who are less experienced. Share your knowledge, offer support, and encourage growth.

Provide constructive feedback: When mentoring, always aim to provide feedback that helps others grow. Focus on strengths, areas for improvement, and actionable steps for growth.

4. Seeking Leadership Opportunities

Leadership isn't always handed to you—it's something you have to **seek out**. While some nurses might have the chance to step into formal leadership roles, others may need to take the initiative to create those opportunities for themselves. Seek out leadership experiences whenever possible, whether it's taking on a project, leading a committee, or volunteering for tasks that allow you to demonstrate your leadership abilities.

Even if you're not in a formal leadership position, you can still look for ways to take ownership of situations, collaborate with your colleagues, and help lead your team. Whether you're managing a shift, overseeing a complex patient care plan, or coordinating with other healthcare providers, every opportunity you take to lead will help build your leadership capacity.

Practical Tips:

Volunteer for leadership roles: If there's a committee, task force, or new project at your workplace, consider volunteering to take a leadership role. This will allow you to practice decision-making, organization, and communication in a leadership capacity.

Take charge of small projects: Leading smaller initiatives, such as organizing a shift schedule or managing a patient care plan, can give you valuable leadership experience.

Take initiative when you see gaps: If there's an area where you think your team could improve—whether it's communication, efficiency, or patient care—take the lead in addressing it. Propose solutions and bring others along with you.

By fostering a leadership mindset in yourself and others, you can create a culture where everyone feels empowered to contribute, improve patient care, and make a positive impact on the healthcare system. Leadership is about inspiring those around you to reach their fullest potential, and in nursing, this mindset can transform not just teams but entire healthcare environments.

CHAPTER 2

UNDERSTANDING THE BIG PICTURE

Nurses are a vital component of the healthcare system—not just as caregivers but also as leaders, innovators, and advocates. Their ability to seamlessly navigate the often-complicated spaces between bedside care and higher-level management gives them a unique power to influence patient care, improve staffing conditions, and contribute to the overall performance of healthcare organizations. Nurse leaders, in particular, play an indispensable role in bridging the gap between the clinical and administrative aspects of healthcare, ensuring that the needs of both patients and healthcare providers are met. In this chapter, we're offering a bit of a "refresher" on the system, helping to clarify just how nurses fit into the larger healthcare puzzle and how their roles extend far beyond the bedside.

Introduction to The Healthcare System Structure: How It Works and Where Nurses Fit In

The healthcare system is a complex web of interconnected players, policies, and processes. At its core, it's designed to provide medical care, treatment, and services to individuals in need. The system operates on multiple levels—from primary care offices to specialized treatments in hospitals, long-term care facilities, and home healthcare. Navigating through this network of providers, insurers, and regulatory bodies requires an understanding of its structure and the interconnections that bind it together. And as a nurse, especially a nurse leader, your role is at the very heart of it all.

Here are the key components of the healthcare system;

Healthcare Providers: The providers are the ones who deliver the care, and as a nurse, you're probably most familiar with their role in your daily work. Here's a quick breakdown:

Primary Care Providers (PCPs): These are often the first point of contact for patients. They address general health needs, provide preventive care, and manage chronic conditions.

Specialists: These healthcare professionals focus on specific areas of medicine (e.g., cardiology, pediatrics, neurology). They're the ones you refer to when a patient needs specialized care.

Nurses and Nurse Practitioners (NPs): Nurses provide essential bedside care, manage medications, educate patients, and collaborate with other professionals to create care plans. Nurse leaders, especially, are key players in both clinical functions and the broader organizational strategy.

Healthcare Facilities

Healthcare isn't a "one-size-fits-all" experience—it occurs in different types of facilities depending on patient needs:

Hospitals: The go-to places for acute care, emergency services, and specialized treatments.

Clinics: These outpatient facilities offer preventive care, manage non-acute conditions, and provide follow-up services.

Long-Term Care Facilities: From nursing homes to rehabilitation centers, these facilities cater to patients with chronic conditions or those who need ongoing assistance.

Government and Insurance Agencies

A lot of the behind-the-scenes action in healthcare happens here:

Medicare/Medicaid: Government programs that provide health coverage for the elderly, low-income individuals, and people with disabilities.

Private Insurance: These organizations offer health plans to individuals and groups, often covering everything from basic care to specialized treatments.

Regulatory Bodies: Agencies like the Centers for Medicare & Medicaid Services (CMS) and the FDA are responsible for ensuring safety and enforcing regulations.

Patients

Let's not forget the central role of the patients in all of this! Their needs, experiences, and outcomes shape the services provided. A patient's journey through the system—from initial contact to follow-up care—impacts everything from resource allocation to healthcare policy. It's safe to say that without patients, the system doesn't work.

The Role of Nurses in the Healthcare System

Now, where do nurses fit into this complex structure? In a word: everywhere. Nurses, particularly nurse leaders, play multiple critical roles, both in direct patient care and at the systemic level.

Direct Care Providers: Nurses are on the front lines, providing bedside care, managing medications, monitoring patient conditions, and working with other healthcare professionals to carry out care plans. Whether it's giving a patient their meds, soothing an anxious family member, or coordinating with a specialist, nurses make it happen.

Patient Advocates: Nurses serve as the voice of the patient, ensuring their needs are met and that they're receiving the proper care. Nurses often mediate between patients and doctors, making sure that the patient's concerns are heard, understood, and acted upon.

Healthcare Innovators: Nurse leaders don't just follow the script—they help write it. Whether it's improving patient care protocols, adopting new technologies, or driving evidence-based practices, nurse leaders are often at the forefront of shaping healthcare policies and improving systems.

So, how do nurses fit into the management side of things? That's where nurse leaders come in. Nurse leaders serve as the bridge between the clinical staff at the bedside and the management team. This is one of the most challenging—and rewarding—roles in healthcare.

Bedside nurses focus on direct patient care, ensuring that individual needs are met.

Management is concerned with resource allocation, staffing models, organizational goals, and financial performance.

Nurse leaders ensure these two groups communicate effectively. They take the feedback and concerns from frontline staff and translate them into actionable insights for management. This way, decisions made at the executive level reflect the realities faced by nurses and the needs of patients. Nurse leaders also ensure clinical staff are informed about new policies, procedures, and practices and understand how they will affect daily operations.

The Impact of Nurse Leadership on Healthcare Outcomes

Nurse leaders don't just manage—they lead by example, and their influence extends far beyond the bedside. The ripple effect of strong leadership is profound and they play a huge part in:

Improving Patient Outcomes: By fostering a culture of safety, implementing evidence-based practices, and prioritizing continuous education, nurse leaders can significantly boost patient recovery rates, satisfaction, and overall care quality.

Enhancing Staff Morale and Retention: A good nurse leader doesn't just give orders—they build a positive, supportive environment where nurses feel valued, leading to reduced burnout and improved job satisfaction.

Facilitating Organizational Success: Nurse leaders also contribute to a healthcare facility's bottom line. By implementing cost-effective solutions, improving operational efficiency, and maintaining high standards of patient care, they help healthcare organizations succeed financially while also enhancing the patient experience.

At the end of the day, nurses are not just caregivers—they're essential to the entire healthcare ecosystem. Nurse leaders, in particular, play a crucial role in bridging the clinical and administrative divides, ensuring that policies, practices, and decisions at all levels align with the ultimate goal: better care for patients. So, if you ever find yourself wondering, "Where do I fit in this big picture?"—the answer is simple: You are the picture.

Bridging the Gap Between Bedside and Management: How Nurse Leaders Make It Happen

If there's one thing that's true in healthcare, it's that the lines between patient care and management often blur. On one side, you have the nurses who are constantly in the trenches—monitoring vitals, administering medications, comforting families, and advocating for patients. On the other side, you have management, who makes decisions that impact staffing, policies, budgets, and overall organizational strategy. So, how do these two worlds meet?

The key player in this dynamic is **the nurse leader**. Nurse leaders are the navigators who steer the ship between these two realms, ensuring that the needs of the frontline staff and the directives of management align. Essentially, nurse leaders are the unsung heroes who ensure that both patient care and the organization's success are thriving simultaneously. Here's how they make it happen:

Advocacy: The Bridge Between Staff and Management

Nurse leaders are often the voice of the bedside staff in executive meetings, making sure that the realities of daily nursing work are understood at the management level. They advocate for appropriate staffing levels, better work environments, and resources that frontline nurses need to provide the best care. At the same time, nurse leaders ensure that the concerns of management are communicated to staff in a way that makes sense for everyone.

For instance, when staffing shortages threaten to impact care quality, a nurse leader doesn't just sit back. They step in to advocate for more support—whether it's pushing for additional hires, promoting shift flexibility, or recommending improvements in workflow. Their job is to make sure that patient care isn't compromised while still aligning with the financial and operational realities of the organization.

Communication: Translating Bedside Needs into Strategic Solutions

One of the biggest challenges in healthcare is ensuring clear communication between the clinical staff and the management team. Nurse leaders excel at breaking down the complex, jargon-heavy world of management and translating it into language that resonates with bedside nurses. Likewise, they take the concerns and feedback from nurses and distill them into actionable insights for management.

Take, for example, a nurse leader noticing that frontline nurses are feeling overburdened with administrative tasks. Instead of simply passing along complaints, a nurse leader will present a solution to management, such as automating some of these tasks or delegating them to other support staff. By communicating both sides' needs effectively, they ensure that the organization can operate efficiently without compromising patient care.

Mentorship: Empowering Nurses While Aligning with Organizational Goals

Nurse leaders also serve as mentors to the nursing staff, providing guidance and support while helping nurses understand the broader organizational goals. This mentorship isn't just about helping nurses grow in their clinical skills, but also about aligning them with the values, priorities, and expectations of the organization.

For instance, if an organization is focusing on improving patient outcomes through evidence-based practices, nurse leaders guide staff to adopt these practices and integrate them into their care routines. This helps ensure that all nurses are on the same page with the organization's goals, fostering a culture of shared purpose. Plus, when nurses feel supported in their personal and professional development, they're more likely to be engaged and committed to delivering quality care.

Decision-Making: Balancing Clinical Needs and Organizational Objectives

Nurse leaders are often involved in decision-making processes that affect both patient care and the business side of healthcare. Whether it's deciding on staffing models, implementing new technologies, or creating policies for patient care, nurse leaders must balance clinical needs with organizational objectives.

For example, let's say management decides to cut costs by reducing nurse-patient ratios. A nurse leader doesn't just accept this decision passively. Instead, they may analyze the situation and suggest alternatives that meet both organizational objectives and clinical needs, such as finding efficiencies in other areas or proposing the use of nurse assistants to lighten the load. In doing so, nurse leaders ensure that decisions benefit both patients and the healthcare system as a whole.

Strategic Leadership: Shaping the Future of Healthcare Delivery

Nurse leaders are not just passive players in the healthcare system; they are often at the forefront of strategic change. Whether it's implementing new technologies, advocating for patient-centered care, or leading initiatives to reduce hospital readmissions, nurse leaders shape the future of healthcare delivery. Their strategic leadership ensures that the system can evolve to meet the growing demands of patient care, all while maintaining efficiency and quality.

In an age of rapidly changing healthcare policies, nurse leaders are essential in steering the organization through those shifts while ensuring the needs of patients and staff remain the top priority. It's their ability to look at the big picture, while still managing the nitty-gritty details of daily care, that allows them to bridge the gap between the bedside and the boardroom.

Balancing Short-Term and Long-Term Goals

In the fast-paced world of healthcare, nurse leaders constantly juggle short-term goals (like meeting daily staffing needs or addressing immediate patient concerns) with long-term organizational objectives (such as improving patient outcomes or achieving financial stability).

By prioritizing tasks effectively, nurse leaders ensure that immediate patient care isn't compromised while also working on initiatives that will improve care in the long run. For example, while they may be addressing an urgent staffing issue today, they're also working on strategies to prevent future shortages or improve nurse retention rates. This ability to balance short-term and long-term goals is essential to the success of both the nursing team and the organization.

In the healthcare system, the gap between bedside care and management can often feel like an insurmountable chasm. But nurse leaders are the essential link that keeps everything running smoothly. They advocate for the needs of frontline nurses while aligning with the broader goals of the healthcare organization. Through effective communication, mentorship, strategic decision-making, and a focus on both clinical and organizational goals, nurse leaders ensure that patient care remains the top priority, even in the midst of complex, ever-changing healthcare landscapes.

The Role of Nurse Leaders in Improving Patient Care and Organizational Success

Imagine a busy hospital floor on a Monday morning. The phones are ringing, patients are calling for assistance, a new admission is being wheeled in, and a medication cart seems to have developed a mind of its own. Amidst the chaos, one figure stands tall—not because they're the loudest or the busiest, but because they have an uncanny ability to bring order to the madness. That's the nurse leader—a combination of coach, strategist, and occasional miracle worker and they hold so many different capacities:

The Patient Whisperer: Improving Care, One Outcome at a Time

Nurse leaders are like the "patient whisperers" of healthcare. They don't just focus on what's happening at the bedside; they look at the bigger picture, ensuring that patients get the best possible outcomes.

Take this true-to-life scenario: A nurse leader notices that a particular unit has been struggling with an uptick in hospital-acquired infections. Instead of playing the blame game, they rally the team and dig into the root cause—turns out, staff had been skipping one small step in hand hygiene protocols during peak hours. With a blend of coaching, humor, and good old-fashioned leadership, they re-train the team, introduce a friendly competition for infection-free days, and reward the unit with coffee vouchers when the numbers improve.

Within weeks, infection rates plummet, patient recovery times improve, and the nurses are cracking jokes about being hand sanitizer evangelists. That's the power of leadership in action—turning a crisis into a win for patients and staff.

The Culture Architects: Building Safety, One Huddle at a Time

If you've ever worked in healthcare, you know that a good workplace culture doesn't just happen—it's built. Nurse leaders are like architects, constructing a culture where everyone feels safe, supported, and valued.

A nurse leader could introduce a daily five-minute "safety huddle" at the start of every shift. It's a simple idea—staff gather, share updates, highlight risks, and offer solutions—but the results are profound. A nurse might mention a patient with a high fall risk, prompting the team to set extra precautions in place. Another might flag a broken IV pump that needs immediate repair, preventing potential delays in care.

Over time, these huddles foster trust and collaboration. Nurses begin to see themselves not just as individual caregivers but as part of a collective mission. And when people work together, amazing things happen—patients get better care, and the team feels unstoppable. Cue the triumphant background music.

The Resource Wizards: Doing More with Less (and Smiling Through It)

Healthcare resources are often as elusive as the last donut in the break room—always in high demand and seemingly in short supply. Nurse leaders, however, have mastered the art of stretching resources without compromising care. Nurse leaders may not perform magic, but their resourcefulness comes pretty close.

Keeping Nurses Happy (and Keeping Them Around)

Let's face it—nursing can be tough. The long hours, emotional toll, and endless demands can make even the most dedicated caregivers feel like throwing in the towel. Nurse leaders understand this, which is why they're committed to creating an environment where nurses feel valued and supported.

One nurse leader made a habit of celebrating small wins. A patient finally mastered their physical therapy exercises? Time to cheer. A night shift nurse went above and beyond to calm an anxious patient? Cue the applause. By recognizing these moments, the nurse leader reminded their team that their work mattered—not just to the organization, but to the people they cared for.

This kind of leadership doesn't just boost morale; it keeps nurses in the profession. And when nurses stay, patients benefit.

Nurse leaders may not wear capes, but they are heroes in every sense of the word. They improve patient outcomes, foster a culture of safety and compassion, mentor the next generation, manage resources like pros, and drive innovation—all while keeping their teams motivated and inspired. Their work is a testament to the fact that great leadership isn't about being in charge—it's about making a difference.

Case Studies: How Nurse Leaders Improved Care Outcomes

Leadership is often best illustrated through real-world stories, where challenges transform into successes under the guidance of effective leaders. Now, Let's look at five fictional but realistic case studies that reveal the diverse ways nurse leaders have elevated patient care and organizational success.

Each of the upcoming stories showcases the profound impact nurse leaders can have, from improving patient safety to fostering meaningful cultural change. Their ability to inspire, innovate, and empower others transforms challenges into opportunities and proves that leadership isn't just about holding a title—it's about making a difference.

These cases would show, nurse leaders don't just respond to problems—they anticipate, strategize, and solve them, creating ripple effects that enhance care outcomes and strengthen the healthcare system as a whole.

Case Study 1: Jessica's Patient Safety Initiative

Challenge:

On the surgical unit Jessica managed, post-surgical infections had become a recurring nightmare. Infection rates were steadily climbing, patient complaints were mounting, and morale among the staff was plummeting.

Strategy:

Jessica decided to tackle the issue with a mix of science, strategy, and a touch of her trademark humor. "Team," she said during a unit meeting, "we're waging war against germs, and I promise you, it's going to be epic." With buy-in from the team, Jessica spearheaded a safety initiative focused on hand hygiene, sterile procedures, and updated post-operative care protocols. She introduced fun incentives, like weekly "Clean Hands, Clear Minds" badges, and provided hands-on training sessions to reinforce evidence-based practices.

Outcome:

Six months later, infection rates had dropped by 30%. Patients were recovering faster, and Jessica's team was glowing—not just because of the hospital-grade sanitizer but because they'd proven they could make a difference.

Case Study 2: Mark's Workflow Revolution

Challenge:

Mark, a nurse leader in a bustling ICU, saw his staff running themselves ragged. Inefficient workflows were causing delays in care, burnout among nurses, and a palpable sense of frustration on the unit.

Strategy:

Mark turned to his team, clipboard in hand, and asked a simple question: "What's the most frustrating part of your shift?" Armed with their input, he implemented a team-based approach to task delegation, restructured shift reporting, and introduced visual boards for real-time updates. "No more guessing games," Mark declared. "Every task has a home, and every nurse has a team."

Outcome:

The ICU transformed almost overnight. Nurses were no longer overwhelmed, burnout rates fell by 25%, and patient care moved faster and smoother. Staff began joking that Mark should moonlight as an air traffic controller.

Case Study 3: Sarah Bridges the Communication Gap

Challenge:

Sarah found herself managing a unit where bedside nurses and hospital management might as well have been on different planets. The lack of communication left nurses feeling unheard and undervalued.

Strategy:

Sarah proposed a novel idea: monthly “town hall” meetings where nurses could share concerns directly with management. She also created anonymous suggestion boxes to capture more sensitive feedback. “This is your chance to be heard,” Sarah assured her team.

Outcome:

The initiative was a game changer. Nurses felt empowered, morale improved, and several suggestions—like updated staffing models and new patient-care equipment—were swiftly implemented. Sarah’s unit became a model for staff engagement across the hospital.

Case Study 4: David's Readmission Reduction Plan

Challenge:

David's hospital was struggling with high readmission rates, particularly among patients with chronic heart failure. Patients were often readmitted due to poor discharge planning and inadequate follow-up.

Strategy:

David introduced a nurse-led discharge planning team, focusing on comprehensive patient education. His team created user-friendly discharge instructions and assigned follow-up nurses to call patients within 48 hours of discharge. "Think of it as a healthcare safety net," David explained.

Outcome:

Readmission rates dropped by 15%. Patients reported feeling more supported, and their health outcomes improved significantly. David's approach was so successful that other departments adopted similar strategies.

Case Study 5: Olivia's Cultural Shift Toward Patient-Centered Care

Challenge:

Olivia worked in a hospital where "patient-centered care" was more buzzword than reality. Nurses weren't engaging with patients as collaborators, and patient satisfaction scores reflected it.

Strategy:

Olivia launched a campaign she called "Listening First." She organized training sessions on empathy, active listening, and communication skills, reminding staff to "see the person, not just the patient." She also started a storytelling board where staff shared moments when patient-centered care made a difference.

Outcome:

Patients noticed the change. Satisfaction scores climbed, and patient complaints dropped significantly. Nurses also reported improved morale as they embraced their role as partners in care.

Case Study 6: Developing a Robust Emergency Preparedness Plan

Challenge:

Nurse Leader Rachel works in a regional hospital located in an area prone to natural disasters such as hurricanes. The hospital has struggled with managing patient care and resource allocation during previous emergencies, leading to delays and confusion.

Strategy:

Rachel conducts a comprehensive assessment of past emergency responses and identifies gaps in preparedness, including unclear staff roles and insufficient supplies. She spearheads the creation of a hospital-wide emergency preparedness plan, incorporating regular disaster simulation training for all staff, establishing clear communication channels, and stockpiling essential resources.

Outcome:

The next time a hurricane hits, the hospital's response is smooth and efficient. Patients are triaged and treated promptly, staff report feeling more confident in their roles, and community trust in the hospital's capabilities significantly improves. Rachel's proactive leadership demonstrates the importance of planning and training in mitigating chaos during crises.

Case Study 7: Addressing Healthcare Disparities in a Rural Community

Challenge:

Nurse Leader Manuel works in a rural clinic that serves a diverse but underserved population. Many patients face barriers to accessing care, including lack of transportation, language differences, and financial constraints.

Strategy:

Manuel partners with local organizations to establish a mobile health unit that provides preventive services and routine checkups to remote areas. He recruits bilingual staff to assist with language barriers and works with a financial counselor to help patients navigate low-cost care options.

Outcome:

The mobile unit reduces missed appointments by 50%, improves chronic condition management rates, and increases patient satisfaction. Manuel's leadership ensures that healthcare becomes more accessible and equitable, highlighting the role of nurse leaders in addressing systemic disparities.

Case Study 8: Creating a Culture of Workplace Wellness

Challenge:

Nurse Leader Priya observes that many nurses in her hospital are experiencing burnout, leading to increased absenteeism, high turnover, and a decline in patient care quality.

Strategy:

Priya develops a wellness program that includes flexible scheduling options, access to mental health resources, and regular team-building activities. She also introduces "wellness rounds," where leaders check in on staff well-being during shifts, and organizes workshops on stress management and self-care.

Outcome:

Over the next year, the hospital sees a 20% decrease in turnover rates, improved staff morale, and higher patient satisfaction scores. Priya's focus on workplace wellness fosters a supportive environment where staff feel valued and empowered, benefiting both employees and patients.

Navigating the Labyrinth: Essential Guides for Nurse Leadership (Because Leading Isn't Always a Bed of Roses—or Even Clean Sheets)

In the high-stakes world of healthcare leadership, every decision carries immense weight.

Nurses in leadership positions understand the gravity of their role and strive to ground their choices in the bedrock of credible, evidence-based information. After all, the well-being of patients and the success of healthcare organizations hinge on their ability to navigate the ever-evolving landscape of best practices, emerging trends, and research-backed strategies. It's not just about keeping the ship afloat; it's about making sure it's sailing in the right direction—and hopefully not into an iceberg of paperwork.

Fortunately, a wealth of valuable resources exists to empower nurse leaders on their journey.

One such treasure trove is the American Nurses Association (ANA) with its comprehensive guidelines outlining the scope and standards of nursing practice. These guidelines, meticulously crafted in the 2021 edition of *"Nursing: Scope and Standards of Practice,"* serve as a compass for nurses at all levels. For nurse leaders, the emphasis on advocacy, ethical practice, and collaboration resonates deeply. The ANA's wisdom extends to specific focus areas like creating healthy work environments (because no one thrives in chaos), fostering effective communication channels (no more "telephone" with crucial patient information!), and cultivating leadership skills through mentorship programs.

Equipping themselves with the right tools is paramount for nurse leaders, and the Institute for Healthcare Improvement (IHI) is a goldmine in this regard.

IHI provides an arsenal of practical tools and resources specifically designed to elevate healthcare quality and safety. Their *"Framework for Safe, Reliable, and Effective Care"* is an invaluable companion for nurse leaders seeking to implement systems-based strategies that enhance patient safety and operational efficiency. Tools like Plan-Do-Study-Act (PDSA) cycles for process improvement and frameworks for reducing medical errors and improving care outcomes empower nurse leaders to translate theory into impactful action—because sometimes, you have to try something new to avoid doing the same thing and expecting different results (we've all been there!).

The connection between strong nursing leadership and positive patient outcomes is a well-established truth, and research provides compelling evidence to support this notion.

A noteworthy study published in the *"International Journal of Nursing Studies"* in 2018 by Cummings et al. sheds light on this vital link. Their findings reveal that leadership rounding directly contributes to better patient satisfaction scores, while team-based care models improve coordination and reduce staff burnout – a win-win for both patients and caregivers (and fewer late-night pizza runs to boost morale).

Regulatory requirements, patient care standards, and reimbursement models are a complex web that nurse leaders must skillfully navigate. Enter the Centers for Medicare & Medicaid Services (CMS) guidelines, a crucial reference point.

These guidelines offer clear direction on aligning organizational goals with value-based care models, reducing preventable readmissions, and improving discharge planning. By leveraging the wisdom of CMS, nurse leaders ensure their organizations stay on the right side of regulations while prioritizing quality patient care (because no one wants a surprise audit—talk about a stressful day!).

While not specific to nursing, the Harvard Business Review (HBR) offers a treasure trove of leadership insights that can be effectively applied to the healthcare landscape.

Topics like emotional intelligence, team building, and conflict resolution explored in HBR articles like Goleman's 1998 piece *"What Makes a Leader?"* equip nurse leaders with valuable tools to cultivate a positive and productive work environment where staff morale and communication thrive.

The future of nursing is brimming with exciting possibilities, and the landmark 2021-2030 Future of Nursing Report from the National Academy of Medicine paints a clear picture of the evolving role of nurses.

This report, *"The Future of Nursing 2020-2030: Charting a Path to Achieve Health Equity,"* emphasizes the critical role of nurse leaders in strengthening interprofessional collaboration, preparing nurses for policy-making roles, and advancing health equity through community engagement. By embracing these key takeaways, nurse leaders become powerful agents of change, shaping a healthcare system that is more collaborative, equitable, and effective.

Continuously engaging with credible resources is the hallmark of a successful nurse leader.

These references not only illuminate the path to evidence-based decision-making but also spark innovative approaches to bridge the gap between clinical and administrative roles. By staying abreast of the latest research and best practices, nurse leaders ensure their strategies resonate with the times, fostering a culture of continuous learning and propelling healthcare forward.

As we conclude our exploration of the healthcare system's structure and the role of nurse leaders, take a moment to reflect on your place within this intricate network. How can you bridge the gap between bedside care and management in your practice? Consider the strategies, case studies, and guidelines discussed here as tools to shape your leadership journey. Reflect on how your current role fits within the broader healthcare system. Identify specific ways you can bridge the gap between bedside care and management in your daily practice.

How can you use your understanding of the healthcare system's structure to improve communication between frontline staff and administration?

What changes could you advocate for to address gaps in patient care or staff support in your unit or organization?

How can you incorporate leadership skills, such as active listening or evidence-based decision-making, to influence positive outcomes in your workplace?

Take a moment to consider these questions and identify actionable steps you can implement to strengthen your role as a key player within the healthcare system.

Pulling Back the Curtain: Seeing the Big Picture

Understanding the big picture in healthcare isn't simply about seeing where each individual piece fits; it's about appreciating the connections and interdependencies that make the system function. Nurses, particularly nurse leaders, are at the center of this intricate web, acting as both advocates for patients and change-makers within organizations. They play a crucial role in ensuring the smooth operation of this complex system.

As we've explored, the healthcare system is vast and multifaceted, encompassing providers, facilities, patients, and regulatory bodies. Navigating this complexity requires leadership that is both compassionate and strategic. Nurse leaders are uniquely positioned to bridge the gap between bedside care and management, translating the realities of patient care into actionable strategies that improve outcomes and foster resilience in their teams.

Key Takeaways

A System Built on Collaboration: Healthcare thrives on teamwork. Understanding the roles of various components and ensuring effective communication between them is paramount for achieving excellence in care. Effective collaboration is essential for optimal patient care.

The Power of Nurse Leadership: From implementing patient safety initiatives to improving workflows, nurse leaders influence outcomes in tangible ways. Their ability to lead with empathy, adapt to challenges, and champion evidence-based practices sets the tone for an organization's success. Strong nurse leadership is a cornerstone of successful healthcare organizations.

The future of nursing lies in embracing leadership opportunities, fostering innovation, and staying adaptable in an ever-changing healthcare landscape. This chapter's insights are a call to action for nurses to recognize their value within the broader system and take ownership of their role in shaping its future.

Self-Assessment

As we conclude our exploration of the healthcare system's structure and the role of nurse leaders, it's time to turn the focus inward. Leadership begins with self-reflection. Consider the following questions to help you connect the concepts we've discussed to your own practice:

How does your current role fit within the broader healthcare system?

Identify specific ways you can bridge the gap between bedside care and management in your daily practice.

How can you use your understanding of the healthcare system's structure to improve communication between frontline staff and administration?

What changes could you advocate for to address gaps in patient care or staff support in your unit or organization?

How can you incorporate leadership skills, such as active listening or evidence-based decision-making, to influence positive outcomes in your workplace?

Take a moment to consider these questions and identify actionable steps you can implement to strengthen your role as a key player within the healthcare system. The strategies, case studies, and guidelines discussed in this chapter are intended to serve as tools on your leadership journey

The healthcare system can be likened to an orchestra, where each section contributes to a harmonious performance. Nurse leaders are not merely players; they are conductors, guiding the performance, addressing challenges, and ensuring that every contribution supports the overall goal of improved patient care and organizational effectiveness.

As we move into the next chapter, "Cultivating a Leadership Mindset," we'll delve deeper into specific strategies for leadership growth and examine the skills nurse leaders need to drive meaningful change. Whether you're a bedside nurse aspiring to step into leadership or a seasoned leader seeking fresh insights, the journey ahead offers opportunities for growth and development.

CHAPTER 3

CULTIVATING A LEADERSHIP MINDSET

Transitioning from a task-focused to a vision-focused mindset is a pivotal moment in the journey of every nurse leader. Think of it as upgrading from a GPS that only tells you where to turn next to one that shows you the entire road map to your destination. While the former gets you through the daily grind, the latter guides you toward something bigger: the long-term impact you want to make as a leader.

Why Leaders Must Think Beyond Daily Tasks

If you're currently in a leadership role, chances are you're no stranger to the seemingly endless stream of tasks: patient care rounds, staffing issues, meetings, administrative paperwork, and the list goes on. We've all been there, buried under a mountain of to-do lists. It's easy to get stuck in the trenches of daily operations. After all, managing the present is essential to keep the ship sailing. But here's the catch: leadership isn't just about keeping things afloat today; it's about steering the ship toward a better future.

To truly lead, you need to lift your eyes from the daily tasks and focus on the broader mission—what's the ultimate purpose you're striving toward? What is the "why" behind the daily grind? When you embrace a vision-focused approach, you start seeing each task as a part of a larger picture. Suddenly, those daily huddles with your team aren't just about filling out schedules—they're about aligning everyone's individual goals with the greater vision of improving patient care, enhancing staff satisfaction, and driving long-term organizational success.

As a nurse leader, you're not just a manager; you're the architect of the future. And to build that future, you need a vision—a guiding light that drives decisions, aligns teams, and fosters innovation. So, the first step is to zoom out from the minutiae of the moment and start thinking about how every action, every decision, contributes to the bigger picture.

Practical Strategies for Transitioning from Doer to Visionary

Shifting to a vision-focused mindset takes practice, but it's absolutely doable. Here are some practical strategies that can help you transform from a task-doer to a visionary leader:

Set Clear Long-Term Goals

Start by defining what success looks like for your team and organization in the long run. What are the bigger objectives that your daily tasks contribute to? Whether it's improving patient outcomes, increasing team engagement, or driving operational efficiency, make sure your goals are measurable and aligned with your vision. As you go about your day-to-day responsibilities, regularly ask, "How does this task bring us closer to that vision?"

Communicate the Vision to Your Team

A vision is only powerful if others can see it too. As a nurse leader, it's essential to communicate your vision clearly and frequently. Bring it into meetings, huddles, and even one-on-ones. When your team understands the "why" behind their work, it creates a sense of purpose and direction. When they can see how their daily efforts contribute to the larger mission, they become more engaged and motivated.

Delegate to Empower Others

When you're stuck in the weeds of daily tasks, you might feel compelled to take everything on yourself. But the best leaders know how to delegate effectively. Empower your team by entrusting them with responsibility that aligns with their strengths. Delegating not only frees up your time to focus on the bigger picture, but it also helps your team members grow and contribute to the shared vision.

A visionary leader doesn't do everything themselves—they inspire and empower others to contribute to the vision.

Schedule Time for Strategic Thinking

In a fast-paced healthcare environment, it's easy to get lost in the daily demands. But if you don't intentionally carve out time to think strategically, you risk being swept up in the operational rush. Schedule regular blocks of time where you step away from the noise and focus solely on the bigger picture. Use this time for reflection, planning, and setting long-term goals. Think about where you want to lead your team and what steps you need to take to get there.

Reflect and Adjust

A vision is not set in stone. As you and your team progress, reflect on what's working and what's not. Are you moving closer to your long-term goals? If not, what adjustments can you make? Regularly assess your leadership approach and make course corrections as needed. A visionary leader is always learning and adapting based on the current realities and evolving needs of the healthcare environment.

Real-world examples would be:

A nurse leader who didn't just review patient care plans—they connected each team member's role to the broader goals of improving patient outcomes and enhancing team collaboration. The result? A more engaged team, better communication, and improved patient satisfaction scores.

Another nurse leader recognized that improving patient care wasn't just about clinical excellence—it was about ensuring that the staff had the support they needed to do their best work. They shifted from simply filling shifts to creating an environment where staff well-being was a priority. By championing a vision of a healthier, more resilient workforce, this leader helped reduce turnover rates, increased job satisfaction, and ultimately improved patient outcomes.

The ultimate goal is to lead with a clear, long-term vision. When your leadership is rooted in a broader perspective, you'll find that your daily actions are infused with purpose and intention. You'll lead with clarity, knowing that every decision—from staffing choices to patient care strategies—contributes to the larger mission. Your team will feel that energy and direction, and they'll be more likely to follow your lead with enthusiasm and dedication.

So, ask yourself: **What is your vision as a nurse leader?** It's time to shift your focus from the next task at hand to the greater impact you can have on your team, patients, and the healthcare system as a whole. Step back, embrace the vision, and start leading not just from the bedside, but from a place of strategic foresight.

The Leadership Trifecta: Resilience, Adaptability, and Continuous Learning

In the dynamic world of nursing leadership, resilience, adaptability, and continuous learning aren't merely desirable traits—they are essential pillars supporting effective leadership. The healthcare landscape is in constant flux, with new policies, technologies, evolving patient needs, and the occasional unexpected challenge. To navigate this complexity, nurse leaders must cultivate these core attributes. Without them, leading in such a demanding environment can feel like navigating uncharted waters.

Resilience: Bouncing Forward

Resilience is more than simply "bouncing back"; it's about "bouncing forward"—recovering from adversity while strengthening leadership effectiveness. It's about weathering the storm without losing sight of purpose or the ability to lead with clarity and conviction.

Resilience is a skill, developed through practice. When faced with challenges like sudden staffing shortages or complex patient cases, resilient leaders remain calm, focus on solutions, and guide their teams. They acknowledge the difficulty but don't allow it to paralyze them. Instead, they frame it as an opportunity for growth and demonstrate strength, perseverance, and hope—qualities that inspire their teams.

Building Resilience:

Reframe Challenges: View difficulties as opportunities for learning and improvement. Ask: "What can I learn from this? How can it make us better?"

Prioritize Self-Care: Leaders must prioritize their well-being to maintain focus and effectively support their teams.

Develop Emotional Agility: Manage emotions and adapt responses thoughtfully. Avoid impulsive reactions; instead, take time to consider the best course of action.

Adaptability: Navigating Change with Confidence

Adaptability is intrinsically linked to resilience—it's the ability to pivot effectively when circumstances change. In healthcare, change is a constant. Whether implementing new technology, adjusting to staffing models, or responding to crises, adaptable leaders navigate uncertainty and guide their teams forward.

Adaptability isn't about blindly embracing every change; it's about recognizing when change is inevitable and facilitating a smooth transition for the team. Resisting change creates tension; embracing it (or at least accepting it) inspires others to do the same.

Cultivating Adaptability:

Stay Informed: Keep abreast of healthcare trends, technologies, and policies to anticipate change.

Foster Team Flexibility: Model adaptability and encourage creative problem-solving within the team.

Maintain a Solution-Oriented Mindset: Focus on solutions, not problems, to empower the team.

Continuous Learning: A Lifelong Journey

In healthcare, knowledge is constantly evolving. From groundbreaking medical breakthroughs that rewrite textbooks overnight to innovative care approaches that redefine patient experiences, the only constant is change. Leaders committed to continuous learning understand this fundamental truth. They recognize that their own growth is inextricably linked to the growth of their teams. By embracing a mindset of lifelong learning, they not only enhance their own expertise but also create an environment where their teams can thrive.

Continuous learning isn't just about attending conferences or accumulating certifications (though those have their place). It's a mindset—a deep-seated commitment to ongoing growth, a thirst for knowledge, and a willingness to embrace the discomfort of learning new things. It's about recognizing that there's always more to learn, always a new perspective to consider. Whether through formal education, the wisdom shared in mentorship relationships, or the invaluable lessons learned through experience—sometimes through hard-won mistakes—continuous learning equips leaders to navigate the inevitable challenges of healthcare with greater confidence and adaptability. Leaders committed to continuous learning not only enhance their own development but also empower their teams' growth.

Continuous learning is a mindset—a commitment to ongoing growth and knowledge acquisition. Whether through formal education, mentorship, or experiential learning, it equips leaders to navigate challenges with greater confidence.

Embracing continuous learning is like building a strong foundation. The cornerstone is a commitment to lifelong education, encompassing formal degrees, certifications, and ongoing training—the essential building blocks of expertise. But a foundation needs support. That's where mentorship comes in, providing the pillars of guidance and wisdom from experienced professionals. The entire structure is then strengthened by fostering a learning culture within the team—the binding mortar that connects everything, encouraging growth, collaboration, and continuous improvement through feedback.

This focus on continuous learning, when combined with resilience and adaptability, creates a powerful synergistic effect. These three traits—resilience, adaptability, and continuous learning—are powerful individually, but their combined effect is transformative, creating a true leadership trifecta.

Resilience enables recovery and sustained focus, allowing leaders to weather any storm.

Adaptability facilitates navigation through change, ensuring that teams can pivot effectively in response to new challenges.

Continuous learning ensures ongoing improvement and preparedness, keeping leaders and their teams at the forefront of their field.

Together, they empower leaders to not only handle challenges but also to lead with confidence, purpose, and grace. This powerful combination can be seen in action in the following examples:

Leading Through Crisis: A nurse leader demonstrated resilience during a severe staffing shortage by remaining calm, reallocating resources, and encouraging creative solutions. By embracing continuous learning, they adapted to a new staffing model, improving team morale and patient care.

Fostering a Learning Culture: A nurse leader in a busy ICU established monthly "learning lunches" for staff to share insights, best practices, and innovations. This fostered engagement, empowerment, and improved patient outcomes.

Self-Reflection: The Inner Compass of Effective Leadership

While continuous learning provides the knowledge and skills necessary for leadership, self-reflection is the crucial process that allows you to internalize and apply that learning meaningfully. It's the inner compass that guides your actions, ensuring they align with your leadership values, goals, and vision. Self-reflection is the practice of looking inward, assessing how your actions resonate with your intentions, and identifying the gap between where you are as a leader and where you aspire to be.

Many nurse leaders, caught in the whirlwind of daily responsibilities, overlook this essential step. They may believe that leadership is solely about action and decision-making. However, without reflection, actions become mere reactions—a series of responses without deeper purpose or understanding. Reflection is the alchemical process that transforms experience into wisdom, turning a manager into a true leader. It's the quiet moment of introspection that allows you to learn not just *from* your experiences, but *about* yourself through them.

Cultivating Self-Reflection: Practical Tools for Inner Growth

Reflective Journaling: The Power of the Written Word: One of the simplest yet most powerful tools for self-reflection is journaling. After a challenging day, or even a successful one, taking a few moments to jot down what went well, what could have been improved, and, most importantly, what you learned from the experience can be invaluable. These written reflections become a personal record of your growth, a goldmine of insights you can revisit and learn from time and time again. The beauty of journaling lies in its honesty—it provides a safe space to examine both your strengths and areas for improvement with fresh eyes, free from judgment.

Seeking Feedback: Uncovering Blind Spots: We all have blind spots—areas where we may not see ourselves as clearly as others see us. Seeking feedback from your team, peers, and even mentors is an essential part of growth. It's about having the courage to ask questions like, "What could I have done differently?" or "How can

I better support the team?" This feedback loop fosters self-awareness, providing valuable perspectives that can help you refine your leadership approach. It's not always easy to hear constructive criticism, but it's essential for growth.

Asking Key Questions: Guiding Your Introspection: Self-reflection becomes more focused and effective when guided by thoughtful questions. Consider asking yourself:

How did my actions today align with my core values and my vision for leadership?

What went particularly well, and how can I replicate that success in future situations?

Where did I encounter challenges, and what specific steps can I take to address them differently next time?

How did my leadership style impact those around me?

Mindful Reflection: Mindful reflection goes beyond simply thinking about your day; it involves pausing to truly understand your emotions, decisions, and interactions. It's about becoming more aware of your internal state and how it influences your leadership. Ask yourself how your leadership style impacted others—both positively and negatively—and how you can adjust your approach to be more effective and impactful in the future.

The dynamic interplay between learning and reflection helps you move beyond surface-level leadership skills to a deeper, more authentic, and ultimately more effective style of leadership—one that inspires your team and drives organizational success.

Self-reflection is more than just a good practice; it's a cornerstone of effective leadership. It enhances decision-making by promoting thoughtful consideration of options, boosts emotional intelligence by increasing self-awareness, and helps leaders stay aligned with their core values and vision. By committing to both continuous learning and prioritizing self-reflection, you transform yourself into a leader who is not only equipped to manage today's challenges but also prepared to evolve and thrive in the face of tomorrow's uncertainties.

The Power of Mindset and Actionable Leadership Growth

A leadership mindset isn't something you're born with; it's something you cultivate, like a garden—sometimes you have to pull a few weeds (bad habits) to let the good stuff grow. Carol Dweck's influential idea that "becoming is better than being" perfectly captures the essence of the leadership journey—it's about embracing continuous evolution.

A fixed mindset, which assumes abilities are static, limits potential. In contrast, a growth mindset encourages seeing challenges as opportunities for learning and development. As a nurse leader, this shift in perspective is essential for navigating the complexities of the healthcare environment and fostering continuous improvement.

When you adopt a growth mindset, setbacks become stepping stones. This approach positively influences not only your own leadership but also your entire team. Leaders who model this way of thinking create a culture where learning from mistakes is encouraged, and where every challenge is viewed as a chance to improve and innovate.

Why Mindset Matters:

Navigating Difficult Situations: A growth mindset provides the mental fortitude to handle challenging situations, whether it's managing a team through a crisis or adapting to new healthcare regulations.

Embracing Change: Viewing challenges as learning opportunities makes you more likely to successfully navigate ever-changing environments.

Inspiring Others: Leaders who embrace growth inspire their teams to do the same, creating a positive ripple effect throughout the organization.

Here's yet another scenario: Imagine a nurse leader whose unit experienced an unexpected surge in patient admissions. Instead of becoming overwhelmed, they focused on clear communication with their team, delegated tasks effectively, and sought input from experienced colleagues. After the surge subsided, they used journaling to reflect on what went well, what could be improved, and how the experience could inform future responses to similar situations. This proactive approach, grounded in a growth mindset, turned a stressful situation into a valuable learning opportunity.

Guided Journaling for Leadership Growth

Now, let's turn theory into practice. Journaling is a powerful tool for fostering a growth-oriented mindset. It allows you to reflect on experiences, assess your leadership style, identify growth areas, and track progress.

Here are some tested and trusted journaling prompts:

How do my daily actions reflect my leadership values?

How do my actions align with my vision for leadership?

What one actionable step can I take today to grow as a leader?

Think of a recent challenge: What did it teach me about my leadership mindset?

What obstacles are you currently facing, and how can you reframe them as learning opportunities?

Reflecting on Growth and Moving Forward

After working through these prompts, consider the bigger picture of your leadership journey. Leadership growth is a series of small decisions, actions, and reflections. Consistency is key.

Remember, becoming a better leader is about progress, not perfection. Regular journaling and self-reflection will help you maintain a continuous cycle of learning, improve your leadership effectiveness, and deepen your commitment to growth.

By combining the power of mindset with actionable steps like journaling, you can foster ongoing leadership growth. This process encourages you to develop a leadership style that is adaptable, prepared for challenges, and deeply aligned with your values and vision. In nursing leadership, the journey of “becoming” is just as important as the destination.

PART 2

SKILLS DEVELOPMENT FOR ASPIRING NURSE LEADERS

CHAPTER 4

COMMUNICATION AND COLLABORATION

When you step into a leadership role, it's like diving into the deep end with a splash of cold water. Everything feels urgent, everything demands attention, and the decisions—oh, the decisions—can be enough to make you feel like you're juggling flaming torches while riding a unicycle.

I remember one of my first real "leadership tests" involved a decision that seemed small but had a ripple effect across the unit. I was asked to address a staffing shortage. The request was simple—reassign a few nurses—but I had to consider the impact. Could we meet the needs of the patients? Would this cause undue stress on my team? And—oh, right—could this possibly mess with the schedule and operations outside of our unit?

In a leadership role, those moments will come quickly, and sometimes you'll need to make decisions in mere seconds. My key guiding principle? Communication. It became clear to me that effective communication—whether with my team, the patients, or the higher-ups—was the linchpin to any successful decision.

Effective Communication: A Lifeline for Leaders

Communication isn't just about passing along information—it's about making that information clear, actionable, and relevant to all involved. It's about being an active participant in conversations, knowing when to listen, when to speak, and how to manage both with a sense of clarity and purpose.

As a nurse leader, your communication spans across a variety of audiences: peers, patients, leadership, and your team. Each of these groups requires a different communication style, tone, and strategy. This doesn't mean you should completely change who you are, but rather adapt and fine-tune how you interact depending on the context.

When communicating with peers, collaboration is key. Nurses and other healthcare professionals work in high-pressure environments, where clear, concise communication can mean the difference between success and chaos. The goal here isn't to dictate, but to collaborate and problem-solve as a team. Be open to ideas, provide clarity when necessary, and remember that each peer brings their own expertise to the table.

Tip: A quick "Can we solve this together?" goes a long way.

Patient communication can be both an art and a science. It's not just about explaining a treatment plan but also offering reassurance, building trust, and helping them feel heard. Patients often remember how they were treated far more than the specifics of their care. This is where your emotional intelligence (more on that later) will be a game-changer.

Tip: Be present. Patients know when you're rushing, and a moment of genuine eye contact can do wonders.

Effective upward communication with leadership is crucial in bridging the gap between bedside realities and boardroom strategies. Here, your communication needs to be clear, evidence-based, and solution-oriented. Leadership often doesn't have the time to dig into the granular details, but they do want to know that you're thinking critically about the bigger picture.

Tip: Be concise, and always bring solutions to the table. A "problem without a plan" isn't a good look in leadership communication.

So, now that we've established the importance of effective communication, let's talk strategies. Developing these skills doesn't happen overnight, but here's a guide to get you started.

Be Clear and Direct: In healthcare, ambiguity can lead to errors. Whether you're communicating a new policy to your team or explaining a complex procedure to a patient, clarity is essential. This doesn't mean you need to sound robotic or overly formal; it just means being straightforward and to the point.

A helpful strategy? The "KISS" principle—Keep It Simple, Sweetheart. Complex medical jargon doesn't help anyone understand better, so break it down.

Cultivate Active Listening: Communication is a two-way street, but many leaders are so eager to deliver their message that they forget the value of listening. Active listening isn't just hearing someone speak; it's engaging with their words, understanding the underlying message, and asking clarifying questions when needed.

If you're guilty of zoning out while someone's talking (we've all done it), now's the time to change that. Active listening builds trust and strengthens relationships—two critical elements in any leadership role.

Use Emotional Intelligence (EI) to Connect: Emotional intelligence, or EI, is the ability to understand and manage your own emotions, as well as the emotions of others. It's a superpower for leaders because it helps you communicate more effectively, resolve conflicts with empathy, and create stronger connections with your team.

Here's the thing—being a "people person" isn't enough. You need to develop the emotional awareness to read situations accurately and respond with the right emotional tone. If your team is stressed or burned out, they don't need a robotic directive. They need understanding and support.

Adapt Communication for Different Situations: The same communication style won't work in every situation. You need to adapt. Think about how you communicate when addressing a high-stakes issue versus a routine task. In the former, you might opt for a more formal, detailed approach; in the latter, you can be more casual and conversational.

Tip: Be flexible. If something doesn't land well the first time, try again, but adjust your delivery.

In the whirlwind of leadership, communication isn't a one-off task—it's a continual process of connection, understanding, and growth. It's the backbone of decision-making, the bridge between colleagues, and the key to inspiring trust and confidence in your team.

By adopting clear communication strategies and honing your emotional intelligence, you'll not only improve your leadership effectiveness but also build stronger, more collaborative relationships. And when the next big decision comes your way—

whether it's about staffing, patient care, or operations—you'll be armed with the skills to communicate it clearly and confidently.

The Art of Listening: It's More Than Just Hearing

Let's start with a little truth bomb—how many times have you caught yourself nodding while someone talks, but you're mentally three steps ahead, planning your next task or thinking about what's for lunch? (Guilty as charged, right?) Active listening goes beyond just hearing words—it's about being fully engaged, paying attention to the speaker, and understanding their perspective.

In nursing leadership, active listening is absolutely vital. It's the difference between hearing a concern from a team member and truly understanding the need behind their words. It's the difference between offering a generic solution and providing one that genuinely addresses the root issue. Leaders who actively listen not only foster a more open environment, but they also **create trust and emotional safety within their teams**.

The Active Listening Framework:

So, how do we actually listen better? It's not about just being "present"; it's about listening with intent and engaging both your mind and your heart.

1. **Pay Attention:** This seems obvious, but it's often where we fail. Give the speaker your full attention, even if it's for just a few minutes. Avoid distractions like your phone, the computer screen, or the urge to finish a task. Non-verbal cues, like maintaining eye contact, nodding, and even leaning slightly forward, can show you're tuned in.

2. **Withhold Judgment:** This might be the hardest part. It's easy to jump into "fix-it mode" or pass judgment on what's being said. But truly listening means withholding immediate responses, especially negative ones, and letting the speaker finish their thoughts. You can always offer your solution after you've fully understood the issue.

3. **Reflect and Clarify:** Use reflective listening to show you're processing what's being said. Phrases like, "What I hear you saying is…" or "It sounds like you're feeling…" can confirm you've understood correctly and can deepen the conversation. Ask clarifying questions, not to interrogate, but to ensure you've got the full picture.

4. **Provide Feedback:** Once you've fully listened, it's time to provide feedback. Be mindful of your tone—remember, you're not just delivering information but fostering a conversation.

Giving thoughtful, considered responses shows that you're taking their perspective seriously.

Professional Relationships: The Heart of Leadership

You've most likely heard this before: "It's not just what you know, but who you know." While this cliché is true to some extent, in the realm of nursing leadership, it's more than just building a professional network—it's about cultivating strong, genuine relationships that foster trust, collaboration, and team cohesion.

Building professional relationships is a key pillar in effective leadership. In healthcare, especially, relationships aren't just about the exchange of information; they're about support, understanding, and shared goals. Strong connections with your team members, colleagues, and even patients create a sense of loyalty and camaraderie that benefits both individual and organizational performance.

But it's not always easy, is it? After all, your job as a leader requires balancing a variety of roles: manager, mentor, motivator, and sometimes even mediator. In a fast-paced environment like healthcare, it can be difficult to find the time to nurture these relationships—but it's essential to do so.

The Foundation of Strong Relationships:

To foster meaningful connections, you need to actively invest in your relationships, both professional and personal. Here's how to get started:

1. **Lead with Empathy:** Empathy is the cornerstone of relationship-building. As a nurse leader, you're constantly interacting with individuals who may be under stress, juggling heavy workloads, or facing personal challenges. A genuine understanding of their emotions and circumstances creates a bond that goes beyond the typical "boss-employee" dynamic.

   For instance, imagine one of your team members is struggling with a particularly difficult patient. Instead of simply offering advice or solutions, approach the situation by asking open-ended questions: "How are you feeling about the situation?" "What do you think would help?" Your empathy demonstrates that you care not just about the task at hand, but about their well-being.

2. **Be Accessible and Approachable:** A leader who is approachable encourages communication and collaboration. Don't hide behind closed doors or work in isolation. Walk the floor, be present during shifts, and check in with your team

regularly. The more accessible you are, the more open your team will be in return.

Make it clear that you are available for guidance, feedback, or even a friendly chat. Sometimes, a simple "How are you today?" can open the door to a deeper conversation.

3. **Show Appreciation and Recognition:** Recognition can be a game-changer in building trust. Acknowledge your team's hard work—whether it's a small thank-you or a more formal shout-out during a meeting. Positive reinforcement shows that you notice and value their contributions, which strengthens the relationship and motivates your team to continue performing at their best.

   For example, after a particularly challenging shift, taking the time to send a thank-you message to the team for their effort can go a long way in reinforcing trust and morale.

4. **Be Transparent:** Honesty and transparency are critical in building trust within professional relationships. As a leader, it's important to be open about the challenges the team faces, as well as any changes that may impact them. When your team understands the "why" behind your decisions and actions, it fosters a sense of inclusion and respect.

If a policy change or a staffing shortage is coming down the pipeline, don't hide it. Instead, communicate it openly, and offer a forum for questions and concerns. This transparency makes you appear more human and approachable, rather than just a decision-maker sitting in an ivory tower.

Emotional Intelligence: The Secret Sauce of Leadership

While active listening is key, emotional intelligence (EI) takes your leadership communication to the next level. EI is your ability to recognize, understand, and manage your own emotions and those of others. When you have a high EI, you become more attuned to the emotional dynamics around you, making you a stronger, more empathetic leader.

As a nurse leader, emotional intelligence is crucial. Every day, you interact with individuals who are experiencing stress, burnout, uncertainty, or fear. Your ability to navigate these emotions—both yours and theirs—can make all the difference in how you communicate, resolve conflicts, and guide your team.

The Role of Emotional Intelligence in Relationship-Building

1. **Self-Awareness in Relationships:** Self-awareness allows you to recognize your own emotional state, which is essential for

relationship-building. If you're feeling stressed or irritable, that can affect your interactions with others. Being self-aware means you can take a step back and manage your emotions so they don't negatively impact your relationships.

2. **Social Awareness:** Social awareness is about tuning in to the emotions of others. If a team member seems off or a colleague is acting withdrawn, social awareness helps you notice these cues and understand their root cause. Once you have this awareness, you can approach the situation with empathy and provide support, even if it's just through a simple "How's everything going today?"

3. **Relationship Management:** In nursing leadership, relationship management is crucial. This is where EI truly shines. It's about effectively navigating your relationships to achieve positive outcomes. Whether it's resolving conflicts, giving constructive feedback, or offering encouragement, a leader who masters relationship management fosters a team-oriented and productive work environment.

For instance, if there's tension between two team members, EI can help you approach the situation in a way that resolves the issue while maintaining respect for both parties. It's not just about diffusing conflict—it's about understanding the deeper emotions at play and offering a solution that satisfies everyone involved.

4. **Influence and Inspiration:** As a nurse leader, your emotional intelligence enables you to influence and inspire those around you. Whether you're motivating your team during a challenging time or inspiring them to take ownership of their work, your ability to connect emotionally with others gives you the power to lead in an authentic way.

Active listening and emotional intelligence are interconnected. The more effectively you listen, the more you understand and empathize with your team. And the more emotionally intelligent you become, the better your listening skills will be, as you tune into the emotions and needs of others.

As a nurse leader, this combination helps you build a resilient, communicative, and empathetic team. You'll be able to guide difficult conversations with confidence, resolve conflicts with ease, and foster a culture of collaboration and trust. When you master both active listening and emotional intelligence, you unlock your full potential as a leader who truly makes a difference.

Practice Exercise:

Practice Exercise: Enhancing Your Communication Skills

Effective listening is a cornerstone of strong leadership. The best way to develop this skill is through focused practice.

A. The next time you're in a conversation—whether in a meeting, one-on-one, or even with a patient—make a conscious effort to truly listen. Try these techniques:

Reflect back what you hear: Paraphrase to confirm understanding.

Empathize with their perspective: Consider their emotions and context.

Respond with awareness and support: Acknowledge their feelings.

B. For the next week, choose one professional interaction each day to focus on building a stronger connection. Use active listening and emotional intelligence to engage meaningfully.

Reflecting on Your Practice:

At the end of the week, take a few moments to reflect:

- What stood out from your conversations?
- Did you notice any shifts in understanding or trust?

- What did you learn about your communication style?

Strong connections are the foundation of impactful leadership. By practicing these skills, you'll strengthen your ability to lead and support your team.

Scripts for Difficult Conversations

As a nurse leader, you'll inevitably encounter difficult conversations. Whether it's addressing performance issues, providing feedback, or discussing sensitive topics like patient safety, these moments are crucial for leadership development. The way you handle these conversations can make or break trust within your team. It can also be the difference between a productive resolution and a situation that lingers in discomfort.

The key to these difficult conversations? Preparation. Just like you wouldn't walk into an exam without studying, you shouldn't enter tough conversations without a plan. The words you choose, the tone you use, and the timing of your delivery can all affect the outcome.

When Giving Constructive Feedback

Providing feedback is one of the most challenging tasks for leaders, especially when you're addressing an area of improvement. However, constructive feedback is essential for team growth and development.

Script Example: "I'd like to discuss your recent shift. I noticed that the handoff communication between you and the night shift was unclear, which caused some confusion among the team. What do you think happened, and how do you think we can improve communication moving forward?"

This approach is open-ended and non-accusatory. It invites the employee to reflect on the situation, thus empowering them to be part of the solution. The key is to focus on behaviors and outcomes, not on the individual.

When Addressing Performance Issues

Sometimes, a more direct approach is necessary when dealing with performance that affects the team's functioning. If an employee's actions are creating a bottleneck or affecting patient care, you'll need to be clear but compassionate.

Script Example: "I've noticed that your response time to patient requests has been slower over the last couple of shifts. Can you tell me if something is impacting your ability to provide care in a timely manner? Let's talk about ways we can support you to improve this."

Here, the approach is empathetic, assuming that there might be underlying reasons for the performance issue. This script also opens the door for the employee to provide their perspective, which fosters a two-way conversation rather than a lecture.

When Discussing Sensitive Topics (e.g., Patient Safety or Emotional Well-being)

Difficult conversations often touch on sensitive topics that require a high level of emotional intelligence. When it comes to patient safety or discussing the emotional well-being of your staff, you must create an atmosphere of trust and support.

Script (For Discussing Patient Safety): "I want to address an incident that occurred during your shift. A medication error was made, and I know this is concerning for both of us. Let's review what happened and identify any steps we can take to prevent this in the future. I'm here to support you as we work through this together."

The key here is to approach the conversation with the intent to support, not blame. Acknowledging the emotional weight of the situation and offering guidance rather than judgment builds trust and fosters accountability.

When Giving Praise and Recognition

Praise is just as important as constructive feedback. It's easy to focus on areas of improvement, but recognizing a job well done is crucial for morale. A well-timed and sincere acknowledgment can do wonders for motivation and engagement.

Script: "I wanted to take a moment to acknowledge the incredible job you did last night. Your leadership during the code blue was outstanding. Your clear communication and quick decision-making ensured that the team stayed focused and that the patient received immediate care. I'm really proud of the way you handled that situation."

Praise, when given specifically and sincerely, can reinforce the behaviors and qualities you want to see more of in your team.

When Incorporating Vulnerability

Another interesting element of effective leadership communication is vulnerability. It can take many forms: admitting when you don't have all the answers, acknowledging your own struggles, or being open about challenges you've faced.

Script (For Admitting Imperfection): "I'll be honest—I don't have all the answers for how we can improve our workflow during peak hours, but I'm committed to finding solutions with all of you. Let's brainstorm some ideas together."

By embracing vulnerability, you show your team that leadership doesn't require perfection—it requires authenticity, trust, and the willingness to work through challenges together.

Now that we've discussed some common scripts for difficult conversations, think about a recent challenging conversation you had with a team member. Reflect on how you handled the situation: Was there a different approach you could have taken? How could you use the scripts provided to improve your communication in future situations?

> *"Vulnerability is not winning or losing; it's having the courage to show up and be seen when we have no control over the outcome."*
>
> *— Brené Brown*

The Role of Vulnerability in Leadership

Given that we've already touched on vulnerability in the context of difficult conversations, it could be powerful to dive deeper into how embracing vulnerability as a leader strengthens communication, builds trust, and fosters a collaborative environment.

As a nurse leader, vulnerability might feel…well, vulnerable. Especially when you're managing a busy unit, making split-second decisions, and addressing both clinical and human challenges. It can seem like you need to project an image of unwavering strength and competence 24/7. But here's the thing: authentic vulnerability can be a surprisingly powerful leadership tool.

Brené Brown, a leading researcher on vulnerability and leadership, has made a compelling case for why vulnerability is essential for building trust, fostering innovation, and creating a safe environment for risk-taking and idea-sharing. It's not about constantly letting your guard down, confessing your deepest fears or admitting every weakness (no need to broadcast your fear of spiders to the entire team). It's about being real, showing up with authenticity, and owning your role in both successes and, yes, even the occasional "oops" moments.

Key Benefits of Vulnerability in Leadership

Building trust is a fundamental benefit of leading with vulnerability. When you're open about your own challenges—whether it's navigating a complex patient case, adapting to a new electronic health record system that seems determined to make your life difficult, or simply admitting you're feeling overwhelmed by the workload—you send a powerful message to your team: "I'm human too." This kind of transparency creates genuine connection.

When your team sees that you're willing to be honest about your own experiences, they're much more likely to do the same. This shared vulnerability creates a sense of camaraderie and strengthens the unit as a whole. Imagine a leader acknowledging after a particularly chaotic shift, "That was a tough one. I know we all felt the pressure, and I want to thank you for pulling together. I'm also going to be thinking about how we can better prepare for similar situations in the future." This simple acknowledgment can go a long way in building trust.

Furthermore, leading with vulnerability fosters a culture of openness and innovation. When team members feel comfortable speaking up, sharing concerns (even if they're worried about sounding "negative"), and offering new ideas—even if those ideas seem a little "out there" at first—you unlock a wellspring of creativity and innovation. This psychological safety is especially vital in healthcare, where new solutions and fresh perspectives can directly impact patient care.

Finally, when you demonstrate vulnerability by owning your mistakes and admitting when you don't have all the answers, you empower your team. This creates a culture of accountability and shared responsibility. It sends the message that it's okay to not be perfect, and that learning and growth are continuous processes. This encourages team members to take ownership of their work and contribute more actively to problem-solving. Imagine a leader saying, "I realize I didn't communicate that change in protocol as clearly as I should have. I'm going to make sure we have a team meeting to go over it again and ensure everyone is on the same page." This kind of ownership builds trust and empowers the team.

Self-reflection:

Think about a recent situation where you demonstrated vulnerability as a leader (or perhaps where you held back). How did it impact your team's trust and communication? Were there missed opportunities where showing vulnerability could have fostered a more open and productive discussion? Reflecting on these questions can provide valuable insights and help you integrate vulnerability more intentionally and effectively into your leadership approach.

CHAPTER 5

CRITICAL THINKING AND DECISION-MAKING

Nurse leaders often find themselves balancing between clinical expertise and administrative duties. It's one thing to make decisions on the floor, where patient care is your main concern. It's another to make administrative decisions that can affect patient care, team morale, and overall operational success. The challenge? We don't always have the luxury of time or all the information we'd like when making these choices.

Think about the times you've been thrust into a situation where patient safety, staff wellbeing, and budget constraints were all in play. One decision, made under pressure, can ripple across the organization, impacting care delivery or even the bottom line.

Clinical reasoning is about using your experience, knowledge, and intuition to make well-informed decisions. As nurse leaders, we need to apply this reasoning not just on the floor, but in administrative settings as well. How can we adapt these clinical decision-making skills to complex situations that don't come with an immediate patient to care for? Here's where critical thinking kicks in.

One technique that works well in these settings is the “STOP and Think” approach. It's simple, but it forces you to pause before jumping into action. **Ask yourself:**

- What do I know about this issue?
- What do I need to know, and where can I find that information?
- Who else needs to be involved in this decision?

These questions are familiar to clinicians who face medical dilemmas—why not use them in leadership? The goal is to apply that same structured approach to the broader challenges you face in your role.

For example, imagine you’re facing a staffing shortage in the middle of a high-acuity shift. It's not just about filling positions; it’s about ensuring the team can still provide quality care without burning out. The “STOP and Think” approach helps you assess the situation, gather necessary information (e.g., who’s available, what shifts are open), and collaborate with others—whether it’s HR, your team, or another department—to solve the problem.

By consistently practicing critical thinking techniques and the STOP and Think approach, nurse leaders can shift from being reactive to proactive in their decision-making. This transition can lead to more thoughtful, data-driven decisions that ultimately improve patient care and staff satisfaction.

Navigating Complex Problems with Evidence-Based for Leadership Success

Leading in healthcare isn't like navigating a straight road; it's more like navigating a complex maze. Decisions are rarely simple, and as a nurse leader, you're constantly juggling competing priorities: patient care, operational efficiency, team satisfaction, and organizational goals. The ability to effectively navigate this maze often depends on using evidence-based strategies—strategies rooted in solid research, proven frameworks, and your own clinical expertise.

At its core, evidence-based decision-making (EBDM) is about using the best available research evidence, your clinical expertise, and, importantly, patient preferences to guide your choices. It's about moving beyond gut feelings or following trends blindly; it's about grounding your decisions in data and a deep understanding of what has demonstrably worked in similar situations.

For nurse leaders, EBDM is transformative. It shifts decision-making from a guessing game to a thoughtful, informed process. Whether you're making decisions about staffing levels, implementing workflow changes, or establishing new patient safety protocols, evidence-based practices offer a reliable compass. By thoughtfully considering research studies, clinical guidelines, and real-time data, you can make choices that aren't just intuitive but are also strongly supported by evidence.

Imagine this: You're a nurse leader in a busy ICU, and you've noticed a concerning trend: an increase in post-operative infections. Instead of simply reacting or blaming it on "bad luck," you decide to take an evidence-based approach. You delve into the latest research on infection control, looking at studies on best practices for wound care, hand hygiene, and environmental cleaning. You also analyze your unit's own infection data, looking for patterns or contributing factors. This data-driven approach allows you to identify specific areas for improvement and implement targeted interventions. Because let's face it, infections are no laughing matter (unless you're a microbiologist with a very specific sense of humor, but don't take my word for it).

Bridging Research and Reality

Integrating clinical research into administrative decisions is a hallmark of effective nurse leadership. It's not enough to rely solely on your clinical experience, especially when faced with complex challenges. You need to look at relevant research that can offer insights into improving operational efficiencies, refining leadership practices, and, of course, enhancing patient care.

Let's say your hospital is considering implementing a new patient monitoring technology. Before jumping on the bandwagon, you could review existing studies and meta-analyses that examine the effectiveness of similar technologies. Does the evidence suggest improved patient outcomes? Has the technology been shown to reduce errors or enhance communication? By blending leadership theory with practical, evidence-based strategies, you make more confident, well-rounded decisions that benefit both the organization and, most importantly, your patients.

Tools of the Trade

Several valuable tools and frameworks can assist nurse leaders in evaluating evidence and making informed decisions. The PICO(T) format (Population, Intervention, Comparison, Outcome, Time) helps structure your research questions and assess how the evidence relates to your specific context. Frameworks like the Iowa Model of evidence-based practice provide a step-by-step guide for implementing new strategies or changes based on research findings.

However, these tools aren't meant to be used in isolation. A truly comprehensive approach involves collaborating with interdisciplinary teams, gathering input from patients and their families, and carefully considering organizational priorities. Evidence-based decision-making isn't just about crunching numbers or reading research articles; it's about integrating insights from diverse sources and perspectives into a holistic decision-making process.

Let's break this down with a real-life example. Picture a nurse leader in a busy emergency department (ED) struggling with patient flow and overcrowding. Instead of simply throwing more staff at the problem (a common but often ineffective response), the leader takes an evidence-based approach. They review current literature on ED capacity management, looking for studies on effective strategies. They discover research showing how specific protocols, such as fast-track systems or rapid triage processes, can significantly reduce wait times and improve patient outcomes.

Armed with this evidence, the leader champions the implementation of a fast-track system in their ED. The results are impressive: wait times decrease, patient satisfaction improves, and staff morale increases as they feel better equipped to handle the patient load. This evidence-based approach transforms the way the ED functions, moving away from reactive, ad hoc decisions and toward a more proactive, data-driven approach.

Think about a recent leadership decision you made that was influenced by evidence or research. What sources did you rely on to inform your decision? How did this approach impact the outcome? Reflecting on these experiences strengthens your ability to use evidence effectively in future decision-making.

Decisions Make Impact

In nursing leadership, decisions aren't just administrative tasks; they're the ripples that spread throughout a unit, a department, or even an entire facility. They directly impact patient care, influence staff morale, and affect operational efficiency. They're the building blocks of your leadership legacy. And just like any architect needs to study blueprints, nurse leaders need to analyze their decisions—both the triumphs and the stumbles—to refine their skills and shape a brighter future.

Every nurse leader has those moments where a decision changes the course of events. Sometimes it's a clinical protocol or a patient care strategy; other times, it's a staffing issue or a budget crunch. But the underlying goal is always the same: to improve outcomes—whether that means safer, more efficient care or a healthier, more collaborative work environment.

Take, for example, a nurse leader grappling with consistently delayed discharge times on their ward. Staff are frustrated, patients and families are anxious, and patient flow is disrupted. Instead of simply accepting the status quo, the leader decides to take a proactive, evidence-based approach. They don't just rely on gut instinct; they gather input from their staff, consult the latest research on discharge planning best practices, and collaborate with interdisciplinary teams, including physicians and social workers. They create a streamlined discharge protocol and ensure everyone—from the nursing staff to the patients and their families—is clear on the new process. The result? Discharge times plummet, patient wait times decrease, and staff feel less overwhelmed. This one decision has a positive ripple effect, improving both patient satisfaction and operational efficiency.

But not every decision is a resounding success. Sometimes, even well-intentioned choices can lead to unintended consequences. Imagine a nurse leader who decides to implement a new electronic health record (EHR) system, believing it will streamline documentation and improve workflow. The idea is solid, but the execution falls short. Training is inadequate, staff resistance is high, and technical glitches plague the system's integration. Instead of the anticipated efficiency boost, the EHR implementation becomes a source of frustration and added workload.

These "oops" moments are inevitable in leadership. The key isn't to avoid mistakes; it's to learn from them. In the case of the EHR system, the leader could have foreseen some of these challenges by involving staff earlier in the decision-making process and investing in more thorough training. Reflecting on what went wrong allows the leader to adjust their strategy, address the immediate issues, and avoid similar pitfalls in the future.

The beauty of evidence-based decision-making is that it provides a framework for both celebrating successes and learning from setbacks. In the case of the successful discharge planning protocol, the leader can use data—post-discharge surveys, readmission rates, staff and patient feedback—to track the impact of the new process. This data-driven approach allows for continuous refinement and even the potential to replicate the successful strategy in other units or facilities.

Similarly, the less-successful EHR implementation offers a valuable learning opportunity. Perhaps the leader can organize focus groups with staff to gather feedback, or research best practices for EHR training and integration. By addressing the challenges and learning from the initial implementation, they can make adjustments that ultimately benefit the organization in the long run.

So, how do you ensure your decisions have a positive impact? It starts with reflection. Think about a decision you made recently that had a noticeable effect—good or bad—on patient care or operations. What steps did you take to ensure the decision was grounded in evidence? How did you evaluate its success or failure? These reflections are more than just mental exercises; they're powerful tools for growth.

Case studies, whether they're your own experiences or stories from other leaders, are invaluable resources for learning and development. By examining past decisions—both the triumphs and the missteps—nurse leaders can identify patterns, build upon successful strategies, and make more informed choices moving forward. It's a continuous cycle of learning, adapting, and striving to make a positive impact on the lives of patients and the well-being of their teams. Because ultimately, leadership is about making those ripples that shape a better future for everyone involved.

Journaling Your Way to Self-Aware Leadership

It's super easy to get caught up in the doing and forget the reflecting, especially in the world of every nurse leader. But one of the most valuable tools you have isn't a clinical guideline or a management framework; it's your own ability to look inward. Journaling isn't just about recording events; it's about holding up a mirror to your decisions, your thought processes, and your leadership style. It's a powerful way to capture lessons learned, track your progress, and refine your practices over time.

Reflection isn't simply looking back; it's about examining your decisions through the lens of growth and self-awareness. Whether a decision leads to resounding success or presents unexpected challenges, taking the time to reflect allows you to understand the why behind your choices, assess their impact, and adjust your strategies moving forward.

As a nurse leader, you're making decisions constantly—from the seemingly small to the significantly impactful. In the rush of daily operations, it's easy to lose track of the thought process behind a particular decision or to skip the crucial step of reflecting on the outcome. Journaling provides the space to pause, to consider your choices in real-time, and to capture the nuances of your leadership in action.

Imagine, for example, you've just addressed a staffing shortage by creatively adjusting schedules. Instead of simply moving on to the next task, take a few minutes to journal about the experience. What factors influenced your decision? Were there any initial hesitations or doubts? How did you communicate the changes to your team, and how did they respond? Reflecting on these aspects provides a wider perspective on your decision-making and highlights areas for potential improvement.

Journaling goes beyond simply documenting actions; it prompts you to explore the why behind your decisions. Did you rely on intuition, or was the decision grounded in evidence? Did you consult with your team, or did you act independently? Writing about these elements helps you identify patterns in your leadership style—patterns you may want to reinforce or revise.

Weaving Case Studies into Your Reflection

Case studies, whether they're your own experiences or stories from other leaders, are invaluable for leadership development. They offer rich material for reflection and analysis. Consider a situation where you had to make a rapid decision during a busy shift—perhaps a critically ill patient arrived, requiring immediate action. What was your thought process as you navigated the situation? Did you utilize evidence-based practices? Were you anticipating potential complications? Did you delegate effectively? Journaling about the decision-making steps, both during and after the event, helps you refine your approach for future high-pressure situations.

Reflecting on these case studies—these snapshots of your leadership in action—can reveal the often-unconscious blend of intuition, experience, and knowledge that informs your choices.

Even those decisions that feel like you were "winging it" are usually rooted in something deeper. Recognizing this builds confidence in your ability to navigate complex situations.

As you consistently reflect on your decisions, patterns will begin to emerge. You'll identify choices that consistently lead to positive outcomes and those that fall short of your expectations. This ongoing reflection is essential for becoming a more self-aware and effective leader. You might notice that decisions made without team input tend to have less desirable results, or that data-driven decisions consistently lead to more successful outcomes.

Perhaps a decision you made early in your leadership journey—one that didn't quite go as planned—shaped your approach to leadership in profound ways. Maybe you took on too much responsibility and experienced burnout. Reflecting on that experience can lead to better delegation strategies and a healthier balance in your leadership.

Through consistent reflection, your leadership practices naturally evolve, becoming more aligned with the needs of your team, your patients, and the organization as a whole. Journaling provides the space to slow down, analyze your choices, and extract valuable lessons from each decision you make. It's not just about writing; it's about becoming a more thoughtful, effective, and self-aware leader.

Consider a recent decision you made that had a significant impact on your team or patient care. Describe your decision-making process. How did you feel about the outcome? What would you do differently next time?

The true power of reflection and journaling lies in their ability to help you make sense of your experiences and accelerate your leadership growth. It's not just about recording events; it's about understanding your thought process, learning from both successes and setbacks, and continuously refining your leadership approach. Every decision offers an opportunity for growth. Your journal is your personal space to explore those moments, gain valuable insights, and ultimately become the leader you aspire to be.

Mini-Activity

I know this may be a bit out there, but this activity is just a step in the grand scheme of becoming way better at journalling. It will help you explore your emerging leadership style by considering how you would handle a common team challenge. Use your journal to record your thoughts and reflections throughout this process.

Scenario (you don't have to use mine): You're a newly appointed nurse in a busy medical-surgical unit. You've noticed that teamwork among the staff seems to be lacking. Nurses tend to work independently, communication is spotty, and you've heard whispers of some minor conflicts. You believe that fostering a stronger team environment would improve both staff morale and patient care.

Instructions:

1. **Journal Entry #1: Initial Thoughts:** Before considering solutions, jot down your initial thoughts in your journal. What qualities make a team effective? What are your values related to teamwork? You can also talk about how the new appointment made you feel

2. **Evidence & Action: In your journal:**

   - List 2-3 specific pieces of information you'd gather to understand the team dynamics.
   - Outline 2 concrete steps you'd take to improve teamwork. Be specific!

3. **Journal Entry #2: Reflection:** After outlining your actions, reflect in your journal:

   - How do your actions reflect your teamwork values?
   - What challenges do you foresee, and how would you address them?
   - What's your next step in developing your leadership skills in this area?

CHAPTER 6

TIME MANAGEMENT AND DELEGATION

"The bad news is time flies. The good news is you're the pilot."

—Michael Altshuler

As a nurse leader, your ability to prioritize tasks in high-pressure environments isn't just important—it's critical. Healthcare is inherently unpredictable. Every shift brings its own set of challenges: patients who need urgent attention, staffing shortages, unexpected crises. Amidst these pressures, effective prioritization is the key to ensuring that you're making decisions that directly impact patient care and team dynamics. But how do you ensure that everything gets done without sacrificing quality?

Let's first start with a little reminder: time flies. The bad news? You can't stop it. The good news? You're the pilot. The reality is that every day brings a new set of challenges, but with the right strategies, you can take control of your time—and that's where prioritization becomes your superpower.

Practical Tools for Time Management in High-Pressure Environments

The key to managing time in high-stress environments isn't about working harder, it's about working smarter. Fortunately, there are plenty of tools to help streamline your efforts:

- To-Do Lists & Prioritization Tools: Use tools like Trello, Asana, or even a simple pen-and-paper list to map out what needs to be done. When you have a lot on your plate, the brain can only handle so much. A visible list gives your mind the space to focus on doing rather than remembering.
- Knowing When to Say "No": As a nurse leader, saying "no" is tough, especially when you feel like you need to be everywhere at once. But learning when to say "no" or "not right now" is key to maintaining your time and energy. Recognize when requests are outside your purview or when they'll distract you from your primary responsibilities. Saying no doesn't make you less of a leader—it makes you a more focused one.
- The "Two-Minute Rule": Inspired by David Allen's Getting Things Done methodology, the idea is simple: If a task can be completed in two minutes or less, do it immediately. This prevents small tasks from piling up and overwhelming you.

But let's get real—tools are only as effective as the mindset behind them. In high-pressure situations, you've got to be able to make decisions fast, and that's where your ability to prioritize becomes your strongest asset.

Delegation

One of the most common mistakes in high-pressure environments is trying to do it all yourself. Nurses are natural caretakers, and as a leader, it's tempting to shoulder every responsibility. But effective delegation isn't just about isn't about relinquishing control —it's about empowering your team to take ownership, use their skills, and contribute to the bigger picture.

However, many leaders struggle with it, often feeling that delegating means losing control over the quality or execution of tasks. The key to successful delegation lies in understanding frameworks that help you balance authority with trust, ensuring nothing falls through the cracks.

When you delegate properly, you're creating an environment of trust and collaboration. One well-known framework is "The 5 Rights of Delegation," a concept commonly used in nursing and leadership circles.

Let's break it down:

1.Right Task: Is the task suitable for delegation? Make sure the task you're delegating is appropriate for the team member's skill level. This includes considering their experience and expertise, as well as whether they have the resources to complete the task effectively. It's about giving your team the tools they need to succeed, not just a to-do list. It should be something that doesn't require your specific expertise but is still important to the team's overall goal.

For example, routine administrative tasks such as scheduling or ordering supplies don't need to be handled by you. But clinical decision-making and situations requiring specialized knowledge? Those should stay in your hands.

2. Right Circumstance: Do you have the resources, authority, and environment needed for successful delegation? Ensure that the circumstances are right for delegation. For instance, if the task is urgent or involves complex decision-making, you may need to reconsider whether this is the right moment for delegation or if it's better for you to take the reins. Understanding the context is key to good decision-making.

3.Right Person: Does the person have the necessary skills and knowledge to handle the task? Delegating to the right person means matching the task to a team member who has the skills, knowledge, and motivation to complete it. Not every team member is suited for every task, so understanding the strengths, skills, and readiness of your staff is key. The best leader knows how to match tasks to the right person. Sometimes, this requires knowing who on your team is not just capable, but enthusiastic about a challenge – and who may need more guidance or support.

4.Right Direction/Communication: Ensure that clear instructions and expectations are set. Clear and concise communication is essential. Ensure that you provide instructions that are both understood and actionable.

Instead of just saying, “Can you handle this?” give specific instructions such as, “I need you to handle X by the end of the day and send me an update at 2 p.m.” When you offer clear direction, you're setting both your team member and yourself up for success. Be specific about timelines, outcomes, and expectations. This step prevents misunderstandings and clarifies your vision for the task at hand.

5.Right Supervision: Delegation doesn’t mean you can just let go and walk away. It’s about offering the appropriate level of supervision and support as the task progresses. The right supervision involves checking in and providing feedback without micromanaging. You don't want to hover over every detail, but you do want to ensure that things are on track.

Make sure your team feels comfortable reaching out if they need clarification or run into obstacles. And when they successfully complete the task, give them credit where it's due. The key here is finding that sweet spot between providing oversight and giving autonomy. Be available for support but resist the urge to take over. Providing feedback – both positive and constructive – helps your team grow and ensures the task is completed to your standard.

When done correctly, delegation can significantly lighten your load while simultaneously developing the skills of your team. You can focus on higher-level tasks like strategic planning, patient outcomes, or innovation, knowing that your team is capable of handling the rest.

However, even with these frameworks in place, delegation isn't always easy. It requires trust, confidence, and a commitment to fostering growth within your team. When you give your team members the space to perform, it shows that you trust their abilities and skills.

In a high-pressure environment, time can slip away before you even realize it. But with the right tools and mindset, you can navigate those busy days without losing sight of what's most important. By prioritizing tasks, utilizing effective time-management strategies, and mastering delegation, you'll not only protect your own well-being but also create a more cohesive, efficient team. Remember that you're the pilot—so, take the reins. Prioritize, delegate, and make every second count.

Urgent-Important Matrix

If you've ever tried to juggle a dozen tasks at once while keeping a watchful eye on patient care, you know that time management in nursing leadership can feel like a high-stakes game of Tetris. The pieces (or tasks) keep falling, and you're left to arrange them efficiently—or risk everything crashing down.

Let's face it: not all tasks are created equal. Some need to be done right now, while others can wait a bit longer. This is where prioritization comes in. The best leaders can quickly identify which tasks will move the needle on patient outcomes or operational efficiency and which ones can be delegated or postponed.

Not everything that feels urgent is important. And not everything that's important is urgent. The classic Eisenhower Matrix (or the Urgent-Important Matrix) can help guide your decision-making in moments of chaos. In this framework, tasks are divided into four quadrants. By clearly identifying which tasks fall into which category, you can make more informed decisions about where your energy is best spent.

SAMPLE EISENHOWER MATRIX FOR A NURSING LEADER

URGENT

NOT URGENT

IMPORTANT

- •Addressing critical clinical emergencies
- •Resolving safety concerns (e.g., incidents involving staff)
- •Managing urgent staff shortages
- •Crafting a clear strategic vision for your team
- •Developing engagement plans that inspire collaboration
- •Mentoring future leaders through coaching sessions
- •Fostering alignment across the leadership team
- •Investing in professional growth opportunities
- •Reflecting on your leadership impact to grow continuously
- •Creating a deliberate and empowering workplace culture
- •Taking restorative, meaningful breaks (yes, they matter!)

NOT IMPORTANT

•Being "on-call" for every minor whim of the team

•Participating in unproductive or surprise meetings

•Drowning in emails and admin tasks

•Wasting time on non-essential paperwork

•Drowning in emails and admin tasks

•Attending meetings with little value or no agenda

•Scrolling social media for "research" (we've all been there!)

•Sorting through emails that don't even concern you

•Engaging in gossip, trivia, or busywork

1. **Urgent and Important:** These are crises or problems that need immediate attention—think code blue situations, or a patient whose condition deteriorates rapidly.

2. **Important but Not Urgent:** These tasks don't demand immediate action, but they are essential for long-term success. Planning your team's schedule, following up with patients, and conducting performance reviews fall into this category.

3. **Urgent but Not Important:** These are tasks that need to be addressed quickly but don't really move the needle in terms of

patient care. Answering non-urgent emails or responding to minor requests might fall here.

4. **Neither Urgent & Not Important:** This category is where you should spend the least amount of time. These tasks are time-wasters. As much as possible, these should be minimized or delegated to someone else.

Balancing Personal and Professional Growth

You've got your professional life to manage, your team to support, and your patients to care for—but what about you? As a nurse leader, it's easy to pour everything into your job, leaving little to no time for personal growth or rest. However, failing to nurture your personal well-being can lead to burnout, which ultimately impacts your professional life.

So, how can you strike a balance between the two? Well, there are four things that have continually worked for me over the past few years; and now, I get to share it with you.

1. Invest in Yourself—It's the Best ROI You'll Ever Get

Just like you expect your team to grow professionally, you must make the investment in your own development. Whether it's enrolling in a leadership course, reading a book on effective communication, or attending a conference, personal growth is a never-ending process. When you invest in your own education and skill development, you not only improve your leadership capabilities, but you also model the importance of continuous learning for your team.

2. Set Boundaries to Protect Your Time and Energy

One of the key challenges of being a nurse leader is knowing when to switch off. Setting boundaries is critical, but it can be hard when you're in an environment where emergencies can arise at any time. However, being available 24/7 doesn't make you a better leader—it makes you an overworked one. Create designated "off" times and stick to them. Trust that your team can handle things when you're not around, and that you'll return with a fresh perspective.

In addition, recognize when your energy is being depleted and take proactive steps to recharge. Regular exercise, hobbies outside of work, and time with loved ones can all help restore balance in your life.

3. Aligning Your Personal and Professional Goals

One of the most effective ways to avoid burnout is to align your personal and professional goals. If your personal values are in sync with your leadership style and work responsibilities, you'll feel more fulfilled and energized. If you're constantly stretching in opposite directions—striving for personal growth while your professional demands are pulling you in the other direction—it can lead to frustration and exhaustion.

Look for ways to merge the two. For instance, if you value family time, can you adjust your work schedule to make that a priority? If lifelong learning is important to you, consider how you can incorporate it into your professional development plan. Finding common ground between your personal and professional lives isn't just nice; it's necessary for long-term sustainability.

4. Know When to Delegate (Again!)

Remember how we talked about the power of delegation earlier? Well, it applies here too. When you take on too much yourself—whether it's at work or in your personal life—you risk burning out. Delegation helps you offload tasks so that you can focus on both your professional and personal growth. Don't try to do it all; trust your team and your support system to help you balance the load.

Striking the Balance—You Can Have It All (But Not All at Once)

In the hustle and bustle of nursing leadership, it's easy to get swept up in the endless demands of patient care, staffing issues, and organizational goals. But here's the thing, like a broken record, once again—you're the pilot of your own journey. Yes, time flies, but you can absolutely steer your ship (or airplane). Balancing your personal and professional life isn't about dividing your time perfectly between work and rest; it's about knowing when to accelerate and when to coast.

Take a moment to reflect: Consider your ability to manage time and delegate tasks effectively. Think about what strategies have worked well for you, and where you've struggled. Have you found yourself drowning in your to-do list, or have you been able to delegate tasks that empower your team? Reflecting on these questions can reveal valuable insights into how well you're balancing your leadership responsibilities. It also provides a chance to identify areas where you might need to shift gears or adjust your approach.

You might not be able to do it all—at least, not at the same time—but you can choose what to focus on, when to hit pause, and when to delegate the heavy lifting. Prioritizing your well-being doesn't just make you a better leader; it makes you a more fulfilled one. And when you're fulfilled, you lead from a place of strength, clarity, and purpose.

So, take a deep breath, adjust the course when needed, and remember that leadership is a marathon, not a sprint. You've got the tools. You've got the mindset. And with a little balance, you've got everything you need to navigate the journey ahead.

PART 3

THE LEADERSHIP JOURNEY—STEP BY STEP

CHAPTER 7

BUILDING YOUR CAREER ROADMAP

If you've ever seen a nurse promoted to a management role, you probably know how the story goes. One day, they're a highly skilled bedside nurse, confident in their clinical expertise. The next, they're handed the keys to the manager's office with little more than a handshake and a "Good luck!"—and just like that, they're expected to lead. No structured orientation. No leadership boot camp. Just a whole lot of sink or swim.

This scenario plays out in almost every hospital unit and healthcare organization across the country. No matter your level of education—whether an Associate's, Bachelor's, Master's, or even a Doctorate—nursing programs teach leadership theory, not the real hands-on experience of managing people, making high-stakes decisions, or navigating hospital politics. Nurse managers quickly realize that leadership in nursing is on-the-job training, often with few resources to rely on.

So, what's the secret to surviving—and thriving—in this transition?

Here's my advice: Find yourself a well-respected nurse manager and ask them to be your mentor. Learn from someone who has walked this path before you. Then, read, read, read—devour every nurse leadership book, article, and resource you can get your hands on. Join your professional nursing organization, build connections, and when the time comes, earn your Nurse Executive Certification (NE-BC) through the ANCC.

Because here's the thing—leadership isn't just about holding a title. It's about growth, adaptability, and creating a roadmap that ensures you don't just survive the transition to leadership, but actually excel at it.

As John Quincy Adams put it, "If your actions inspire others to dream more, learn more, do more, and become more, you are a leader." But before you can inspire others, you need to invest in your own growth. Let's get started.

Setting SMART Goals for Leadership Success

Every great leader starts with a vision – a clear picture of where they want to go and a plan to get there. But in nursing leadership, it's easy to get swept up in the daily demands and lose sight of the bigger picture. It's like being handed the keys to a car without a map – you might know how to drive, but you're not sure where you're headed. If you don't actively shape your career development, you risk reacting to circumstances instead of leading with intention.

That's where the power of goal setting comes in This is where goal-setting becomes crucial. Not just vague aspirations like "I want to be a great leader," but SMART goals—Specific, Measurable, Achievable, Relevant, and Time-bound.

- **Specific:** A specific goal is clear and well-defined. It answers the questions of who, what, where, when, why, and how. Instead of "Improve my communication skills," a specific goal would be "Implement monthly one-on-one check-ins with each staff member to improve team communication and engagement."
- **Measurable:** A measurable goal allows you to track your progress and know when you've achieved it. Instead of "Learn more about leadership," a measurable goal would be "Complete the 'Leading Through Change' workshop and receive a certificate of completion."
- **Achievable:** An achievable goal is realistic and attainable given your current resources and constraints. It should stretch you slightly but not be so far out of reach that it becomes discouraging.
- **Relevant:** A relevant goal aligns with your overall career aspirations and values. It should be something that truly matters to you and contributes to your long-term vision.

•**Time-bound:** A time-bound goal has a deadline. This creates a sense of urgency and helps you stay focused. Instead of "Get certified someday," a time-bound goal would be "Obtain the Nurse Executive Certification (NE-BC) within the next three years."

SMART goals are the GPS coordinates that guide you on your leadership journey. They provide direction, motivation, and a way to measure your success.

Short-Term Goals: Building Momentum

Think of short-term goals as the mile markers on your leadership roadmap. They're the smaller, achievable steps that build momentum and propel you forward. They're also a chance to experiment and see what kind of leader you want to be. Maybe you want to get better at public speaking. A short-term goal could be to volunteer to present at your unit's next staff meeting. Or maybe you want to improve your ability to delegate tasks. You could set a short-term goal to delegate at least two tasks a week to members of your team. Perhaps you've identified a need to enhance your skills in leading through change.

A relevant short-term goal might be to enroll in a "Leading Through Change" workshop within the next three months, committing to actively participating in all modules. Or maybe you recognize the importance of stronger communication within your team. You could aim to implement monthly one-on-one check-ins with each staff member for the next six months, dedicating specific times for these conversations. Expanding your professional network is also a valuable short-term goal. Consider joining the American Nurses Association within the next month and making it a point to attend a local chapter meeting within the next six months, connecting with at least three other nurse leaders.

Long-Term Goals: Defining Your Leadership Legacy

Long-term goals are your destination – the vision of where you want to be as a leader. They're about defining your impact and the legacy you want to leave. Maybe you dream of becoming a Chief Nursing Officer. Or perhaps you're passionate about influencing healthcare policy at a national level. These long-term goals provide direction and motivation. Perhaps you envision yourself as a highly respected nurse executive.

A long-term goal aligned with this vision could be to obtain the Nurse Executive Certification (NE-BC) within the next three years, demonstrating your advanced leadership competency. Or maybe you see yourself leading a team of nurses as a director of nursing. A relevant long-term goal might be to transition from nurse manager to this director role within the next five years, focusing on gaining experience in budget management and strategic planning to prepare yourself. For those with a passion for broader healthcare impact, contributing to healthcare policy could be a significant long-term goal. This might involve joining a local or state nursing policy committee within the next year, actively participating in meetings, and contributing to policy recommendations.

The Power of a Written Plan: Turning Dreams into Reality

A goal without a written plan is just a wish. It's like knowing you want to go to the beach but not knowing which roads to take. Writing down your goals is a crucial step – studies show that people who do so are significantly more likely to achieve them. It makes the goal tangible and reinforces your commitment. Break down your goals into smaller, actionable steps. Set deadlines for each step. And track your progress – celebrate the small wins along the way!

As Warren Bennis wisely said, "Leadership is the capacity to translate vision into reality." Your career roadmap isn't just about climbing the ladder; it's about intentionally shaping your leadership path. It's about becoming the leader you aspire to be.

Formal Education and Certifications in Nursing Leadership

In nursing, clinical expertise gets you through the door, but leadership expertise keeps you in the room. Yet, many nurse leaders find themselves promoted without the formal training or credentials that make leadership easier to navigate. Suddenly, you're expected to manage budgets, lead teams, and navigate complex policies—all without a structured foundation. Sound familiar?

While experience is invaluable, formal education and certifications provide the structured knowledge and credibility that can set you apart. A degree or certification won't magically make you a great leader overnight, but it equips you with tools to make better decisions, advocate effectively, and stay ahead in a rapidly evolving healthcare landscape.

If you're serious about advancing in leadership, pursuing a higher degree can provide strategic advantages. Here's a quick breakdown:

- Bachelor of Science in Nursing (BSN) – A stepping stone for leadership; often required for management roles.

•Master of Science in Nursing (MSN) – Leadership or Administration Focus – Provides deeper knowledge in healthcare systems, finance, and management.

•Doctor of Nursing Practice (DNP) – Executive Leadership Track – A terminal degree that positions you for C-suite roles, policy influence, and large-scale organizational change.

•MBA in Healthcare Management – Ideal if you want a strong business and financial foundation alongside leadership.

While pursuing a degree requires time and financial investment, many healthcare organizations offer tuition reimbursement or scholarship opportunities. If formal education isn't feasible now, consider certifications as a more immediate step.

Here are some key certifications that help to validate your expertise and commitment to leadership. Some of the most recognized ones include: NE-BC (Nurse Executive Board Certification), CENP (Certified in Executive Nursing Practice), FACHE (Fellow of the American College of Healthcare Executives), CNL (Clinical Nurse Leader Certification), and CNML (Certified Nurse Manager & Leader).

Many nurses delay pursuing certifications because they feel they're "not ready." The reality? You'll never feel 100% ready—but starting now means you'll be prepared when opportunity knocks.

Education Alone Isn’t Enough—But It Opens Doors. It’s a stepping stone, not a silver bullet. Let's be clear: a degree or certification alone won't magically transform you into a leadership guru. Real-world leadership experience is invaluable—it's where you learn to navigate the messy, unpredictable realities of managing teams and making critical decisions under pressure.

However, in today's competitive healthcare landscape, education provides a crucial strategic advantage. It's not just about checking a box; it signals to potential employers that you're serious about leadership, that you're invested in your professional growth. It exposes you to new ideas, expands your network, and builds confidence in your decision-making abilities. It gives you a solid foundation upon which to build your practical experience.

As John Quincy Adams wisely stated, “If your actions inspire others to dream more, learn more, do more, and become more, you are a leader.” Education, combined with practical experience and self-reflection, empowers you to become that kind of leader. It gives you the tools and knowledge to inspire, innovate, and make a real difference. It's not simply about being more qualified; it's about being more effective. The question isn't if you should pursue further education, but what your next step will be on your path to leadership.

Leveraging Mentorship and Coaching

If leadership is a journey, then mentorship is your best shortcut. The truth is, no leader—no matter how skilled—rises to success alone. Behind every confident, competent nurse leader is usually a mentor who helped shape their path.

Yet, many new nurse managers struggle in silence, afraid to admit they feel lost. They tell themselves, "I should know this already," or "I'll figure it out on my own." But leadership isn't an individual sport—it's a team effort. And having the right mentor can mean the difference between thriving and merely surviving.

Think about it: No matter how many books you devour or certifications you earn, nothing truly prepares you for the nitty-gritty reality of leadership like experience. But experience takes time – years, sometimes decades. A mentor acts as a shortcut, giving you access to their hard-earned wisdom, saving you from having to make every single mistake yourself. They've walked the path you're now on, and they can offer insights you won't find in any textbook.

A great mentor will:

- Offer guidance when you're navigating tricky situations (like that time you had to deal with a scheduling conflict involving three nurses and a patient with a last-minute emergency).

•Challenge you to think bigger and push beyond your comfort zone (like suggesting you present at a conference, even though public speaking makes your palms sweat).

•Provide honest feedback, even when it's tough to hear (because sometimes, you need someone to tell you that your communication style could use some tweaking).

•Help you avoid the pitfalls they encountered on their own journey (like that budget blunder they made early in their career, which they can now help you avoid).

Finding the right mentor is like finding the right hiking buddy – you need someone whose pace and style match yours. It's not just about finding someone in a leadership position; it's about finding someone whose leadership style you admire and whose values resonate with your own.

Look for these key qualities:

Experience: They've walked the path you're on and have a proven track record of success.

Approachability: They're willing to share their knowledge without ego and make you feel comfortable asking questions.

Honesty: They'll give you the straight truth, even when it's uncomfortable, because they genuinely want to help you grow.

Commitment: Mentorship is a two-way street; they're willing to invest their time and energy in your development.

So where do you find this mentor?

Well, you've got to start within your own organization. Identify a respected nurse manager or executive whose leadership you admire and reach out for an informal chat. Professional organizations like the American Nurses Association (ANA) and the American Organization for Nursing Leadership (AONL) often have mentorship programs. And if in-person mentorship isn't feasible, explore virtual coaching programs or online leadership forums.

Mentorship vs. Coaching—Two Sides of the Same Coin

While people often use the terms interchangeably, mentorship and coaching serve different purposes. Think of mentorship as a long-term relationship focused on your overall career growth, while coaching is a shorter-term engagement focused on developing specific skills.

A mentor offers wisdom and guidance based on their own experiences, while a coach provides tools and strategies to help you overcome specific challenges. Ideally, having both in your corner would be beneficial. If you're struggling with a particular issue (like conflict resolution or time management), a coach might be the best option. If you're looking for long-term career advice and leadership insights, a mentor is the way to go.

Simply having a mentor isn't enough; you need to be an active participant in the relationship. Before meeting with your mentor, identify the specific challenges you're facing and what you hope to gain from the interaction. Are you struggling with confidence? Delegation? Work-life balance? Come prepared with specific questions or topics you'd like to discuss. Respect their time by being punctual and making the most of your meetings. And most importantly, follow through on their advice. Show them you value their insights by acting on their recommendations. Be open to feedback, even when it's constructive criticism. Remember, a mentor isn't there to tell you what you want to hear; they're there to help you grow.

Let's take a look at Maria's story, a nurse who transitioned into a leadership role without guidance or preparation.

Maria had been a bedside nurse for eight years when she was promoted to nurse manager. She was thrilled about the opportunity, but quickly felt overwhelmed by the new responsibilities. She was suddenly in charge of scheduling, budgeting, and handling staff conflicts – things she hadn't been trained for. She started dreading work and questioning her career choice. Then, she connected with a senior nurse leader, someone she admired, and asked for guidance. This leader agreed to mentor her.

Over the next year, they met regularly, discussing everything from difficult conversations to leading with confidence. With her mentor's support, Maria developed a clear leadership style, learned how to set boundaries, and became a strong advocate for her team. She not only thrived in her role but eventually became a mentor herself, paying it forward to the next generation of nurse leaders.

Beyond a single mentor, building a strong support network is essential. Surround yourself with people who challenge you to grow, inspire you with their work ethic and vision, and offer diverse perspectives on leadership. This network could include colleagues, fellow nurse leaders, online communities, or leadership groups. The more diverse your network, the better equipped you'll be to navigate the challenges of leadership.

Mentorship is fundamentally about leadership – helping others become the best versions of themselves. If you're serious about excelling in your career, seek out mentors who can guide you on your path, and be a mentor to others when you have the opportunity. As Ralph Nader wisely said, "The function of leadership is to produce more leaders, not more followers." Who will you learn from? And more importantly, who will you help rise?

Joining a Professional Organization (It's More Than Just Free Pens)

Stepping into leadership is like stepping into a new world—one filled with exciting possibilities, but also new challenges, expectations, and, let's be honest, some unspoken rules that can feel a bit mysterious. The good news is; you don't have to navigate this new terrain alone.

If mentorship provides invaluable one-on-one guidance, then professional organizations offer a whole ecosystem of support, knowledge, and opportunities—your professional tribe. These organizations aren't just for networking (though that's a definite perk); they're a goldmine of resources that can significantly accelerate your leadership journey.

Too often, nurses view professional organizations as an optional "extra"—a nice-to-have but not a necessity. This is a missed opportunity. They are one of the most powerful tools available for career advancement and leadership development. Here's what membership in the right organization can do for you:

Access to Exclusive Leadership Programs: Many organizations offer workshops, training programs, and leadership development courses designed specifically for nurse leaders. These programs provide targeted training on the skills you need to excel, from strategic planning to conflict resolution.

•Networking with the Best: Connect with established leaders, potential mentors, and like-minded peers. These connections can open doors to new career opportunities, provide valuable insights, and offer a supportive community.

- **Advocacy and Influence:** Be part of the policy discussions that shape the future of nursing and healthcare. Your voice can help influence staffing policies, healthcare laws, and patient care standards.
- **Certifications & Continuing Education:** Stay ahead of the curve with access to certification programs, conferences, and exclusive research. This ensures you're always learning and growing.
- **Job Opportunities & Career Advancement:** Many organizations post leadership positions before they're widely advertised, giving members a significant advantage in the job market.

Not all nursing organizations are created equal. If you're serious about developing your leadership skills, consider these powerhouse groups:

- **American Nurses Association (ANA):** The ANA is the largest professional nursing organization in the U.S., offering a wide range of resources, including leadership training, policy advocacy, and career development tools. Their Leadership Institute is a structured program designed to enhance skills at all career stages, and their involvement in policy and advocacy allows you to shape the future of nursing. Plus, ANA members often get discounts on certifications, like the NE-BC.

- **American Organization for Nursing Leadership (AONL):** If you're aiming for senior leadership roles, AONL is a must. It focuses specifically on nurse executives, directors, and managers, offering intensive training programs for emerging leaders and providing unparalleled networking opportunities with CEOs, CNOs, and other top healthcare executives. They also provide access to exclusive research and industry reports, keeping you at the forefront of leadership and management strategies.
- **American Association of Critical-Care Nurses (AACN):** For those in critical care, AACN provides specialized leadership training tailored to the unique demands of high-intensity environments like ICUs and ERs. They also offer scholarships and grants for leadership certifications and continuing education, and provide access to some of the best minds in critical-care nursing leadership through conferences and mentorship programs.
- **State & Specialty Nursing Associations**: Don't overlook the power of local connections! Many states and specialties have their

own leadership groups that provide localized resources, mentorship programs, and targeted networking opportunities. Check with your state's nursing board or look into specialty groups like the Emergency Nurses Association (ENA) or Oncology Nursing Society (ONS).

In the business world, an MBA can signal leadership potential. In nursing, certifications serve a similar purpose, demonstrating your commitment to professional development and expertise in leadership and management.

The two most respected nurse leadership certifications are:

- **Nurse Executive Certification (NE-BC):** Offered by the ANCC, this certification is ideal for nurse managers, directors, and executives, covering key areas like finance, human resources, and strategic leadership. It requires two years of leadership experience and an active RN license.

- **Certified Nurse Manager & Leader (CNML):** Offered by AONL, this certification focuses on operational leadership, team management, and patient-centered care. It's ideal for new or aspiring nurse managers and requires one year of leadership experience and an active RN license.

These certifications not only boost your resume but also demonstrate your dedication to leadership excellence and can increase your earning potential.

Becoming a great nurse leader isn't about figuring everything out on your own. It's about learning from those who've already walked the path, and professional organizations provide direct access to that collective wisdom.

So, what's your next step? Maybe it's exploring the ANA's Leadership Institute, or perhaps it's finally registering for that AONL conference you've been eyeing. Or maybe it's simply reaching out to a local chapter of your specialty nursing association. Whatever it is, take that first step. Your leadership journey is just beginning—and you don't have to take it alone.

CHAPTER 8

TRANSITIONING FROM BEDSIDE TO LEADERSHIP ROLES

As always, I'll be making an analogy to start this out. Imagine a seed. It holds within it the potential to become a mighty oak, but it needs the right conditions to grow: sunlight, water, fertile soil. Kevin was like that seed. He had the potential for leadership, but he needed to cultivate the right skills, the right mindset, and the right approach to unlock it. Kevin stared at the blinking cursor on his laptop screen, a blank resume template mocking his ambition. He'd envisioned this moment so differently: confidently striding into interviews, effortlessly charming recruiters, landing the leadership role he craved. The reality, however, was a gnawing sense of inadequacy. He was a nurse, yes, a damn good one, but a leader? The thought felt both exhilarating and terrifying. He knew he had the potential, the drive, the quiet fire in his belly, but translating that into a resume, into interview answers, into tangible action – that was the challenge.

Applying for leadership positions can feel like climbing Everest in flip-flops. It's daunting, it's competitive, and it's easy to get discouraged. But the secret, Kevin realized, wasn't some magic formula or hidden handshake. It was a shift in perspective. He wasn't just a nurse administering medications; he was a strategist coordinating complex patient care, a problem-solver navigating unexpected crises, an advocate ensuring his patients received the best possible treatment. Leadership, he understood, wasn't about titles or corner offices; it was about influence, about impact, about inspiring others to be their best. And that was something he could absolutely do.

A strong leadership resume should include:

•**A compelling summary**: One or two sentences that capture your leadership potential and vision.

•**Quantifiable achievements:** Numbers help. For example: "Spearheaded the implementation of a new medication tracking system, resulting in a 20% reduction in medication errors within the first quarter."

•**Relevant skills:** Budget management, staff training, conflict resolution—if you've done it, list it.

•**Professional development:** Leadership workshops, certifications, and committee involvement show initiative.

Now, back to Kevin. His first task was the resume. Most nursing resumes, Kevin knew, were a litany of duties performed, not results achieved. His had to be different. It had to whisper, no, shout "leadership." Instead of listing "administered medications," he wrote "Implemented a new medication administration protocol that reduced patient wait times by 15%." Instead of "assisted with patient care," he highlighted "Mentored three new nurses, fostering their professional development and contributing to a 20% improvement in team morale." He quantified his achievements whenever possible, using data to showcase the positive impact he'd made. His resume wasn't just a list of tasks; it was a testament to his leadership in action.

The interview loomed next, a formidable beast. Kevin knew the interviewers weren't looking for perfection; they were searching for potential. They wanted to see confidence, yes, but also humility. They wanted to see vision, but also practicality. They wanted to see someone who could inspire a team, navigate conflict, and make tough decisions under pressure. He prepared for the inevitable "Tell me about a time..." questions, crafting stories that showcased his problem-solving skills, his ability to build consensus, and his unwavering focus on patient care. He even practiced his answers in the mirror, fine-tuning his delivery until he felt confident, but not cocky. He knew a little humor could go a long way – "Well, there was that time the power went out during a critical surgery, and we had to rely on flashlights and sheer ingenuity..." – but he also knew the importance of pivoting quickly to the substantive example and the positive outcome.

Networking, the final piece of the puzzle, felt the most daunting. Kevin wasn't a natural schmoozer. The thought of awkward small talk at conferences made his palms sweat. But he realized networking wasn't about selling himself; it was about building genuine connections. He started small, reconnecting with former colleagues, joining a professional nursing association, and even updating his LinkedIn profile. He discovered that networking was less about asking for favors and more about sharing experiences, offering support, and building relationships. He found a mentor, a seasoned nurse leader who offered guidance, shared insights, and opened doors to new opportunities.

Kevin walked into his leadership interview not with a feeling of complete readiness, but with a quiet confidence. He knew he had the skills, the experience, and the mindset to grow into the role. He understood that leadership wasn't a destination; it was a journey. And he was ready to begin. He didn't get the job that day, but he learned from the experience, polished his approach, and kept moving forward. His journey was unique, and he was ready to embrace it.

Kevin's experience, though imagined, resonates with the experiences of many. It reminds us that the path to leadership isn't always smooth, but it's always possible. The lessons he learned – about reframing our narratives, showcasing our strengths, and building meaningful relationships – are applicable to us all. So, take a moment to reflect on your own journey. What steps can you take today to move closer to your leadership goals? Your potential is there, waiting to be unleashed.

Common Challenges When Stepping Into a Management Role

Stepping into a leadership role as a nurse can feel a bit like showing up to your first day at a new job—only to find out you're the boss. Suddenly, the people you used to share coffee breaks with are looking to you for decisions, and those tough calls you once grumbled about? Now, they're yours to make. The transition is exciting, but it's also full of unexpected hurdles. Here's what to expect and how to navigate the shift with confidence.

1. **From Peer to Leader:** One day, you're laughing in the break room with your colleagues. The next, you're the one approving their PTO requests and giving performance feedback. It can be tough to redefine relationships, especially when you're managing former peers. Some may be thrilled for you, while others might be skeptical (or even a little resentful). The key is

balance—maintaining camaraderie while setting clear professional boundaries. You're still you, but with added responsibilities. Approach the shift with transparency, fairness, and a willingness to listen.

2. **Decision-Making Pressure:** As a bedside nurse, you relied on protocols and teamwork. Now, you'll need to make judgment calls that impact both patient care and team dynamics. It's not uncommon to second-guess yourself at first, but trust that your clinical experience has prepared you more than you realize. When in doubt, lean on mentors, gather input, and remember—decisiveness is a skill that gets sharper with practice.

3. **Conflict Management:** Welcome to leadership—where "putting out fires" is a daily sport. Disagreements between staff, scheduling conflicts, and navigating workplace tensions are now part of your reality. The best leaders handle conflict with a mix of fairness, active listening, and a dash of diplomacy. Pro tip: Never make big decisions when emotions are running high. Give people space to cool off, gather perspectives, and address issues head-on with solutions, not blame.

4. **The "Too Many Hats" Dilemma:** Nurse leaders are part clinician, part administrator, part motivator, and—on particularly chaotic days—part magician. You'll be expected to

juggle patient care priorities, team morale, budgeting concerns, and compliance requirements, sometimes all before lunch. The trick? Prioritization. Learn to delegate, manage your time wisely, and accept that you can't do it all alone. Find efficiencies where you can, and don't hesitate to tap into the strengths of your team.

5. **Self-Doubt and Growing Pains:** It's natural to feel out of your depth at times. Many new nurse-leaders experience "imposter syndrome," that nagging voice that whispers, "Are you really ready for this?" Spoiler alert: You are. Growth comes with discomfort, and every great leader has had moments of doubt. The key is to keep learning, seek mentorship, and remind yourself that leadership isn't about knowing everything—it's about being willing to learn, adapt, and uplift those around you.

Transitioning into a leadership role isn't just about a new job title—it's about evolving into a guide, a decision-maker, and a source of support for your team. The challenges are real, but so is your ability to tackle them. Embrace the learning curve, laugh at the awkward moments, and take it one day at a time. Up next: Imposter syndrome—why every leader faces it and how to manage it without losing your sanity.

Managing Imposter Syndrome in New Roles

Stepping into a leadership role often triggers a silent, nagging question: "Am I really qualified for this?" This self-doubt, often called imposter syndrome, is a common experience, especially in nursing, where the transition from bedside care to management can feel like navigating uncharted territory. It's easy to feel like you're faking it, even when you've earned your place. But here's the truth: leadership isn't about having all the answers; it's about guiding a team, making informed decisions, and adapting to the inevitable challenges. Your strong foundation of clinical experience and honed problem-solving skills are the bedrock of effective leadership—recognizing this helps reframe self-doubt as a natural part of growth, not a sign of inadequacy.

So, how do you tame that imposter voice and step into your leadership potential with confidence? It starts with practical strategies. Keep a running record of your professional achievements, positive feedback from colleagues, and moments of success, no matter how small. This tangible evidence reinforces your competence and combats the tendency to minimize your accomplishments. Seeking mentorship from experienced leaders is invaluable. They can offer perspective, share their own "I had no idea what I was doing at first" stories (and we all have them!), and provide reassurance when self-doubt creeps in. Regular self-check-ins are crucial. Distinguish between a legitimate knowledge gap, which can always be addressed through learning and development, and the unfounded whispers of imposter syndrome.

Remember, leadership is a continuous learning process. No one, not even the most seasoned executive, starts with all the answers, and no leader operates in isolation. Embrace this journey of growth, be open to feedback (even the constructive kind), and lean on your supportive network. These actions can transform self-doubt into self-assurance. Recognize that you're not alone in this—most leaders, at some point, have felt like they were faking it. The key is to reframe your thinking. Instead of viewing leadership as a fixed destination you should have already reached, see it as an evolving skillset, just like nursing was when you first began. Just as you grew and developed your clinical skills, you will grow and develop your leadership skills. Here are some practical strategies to help you on your way:

Remember why you were chosen: Your skills, experience, and judgment earned you this role—trust the process and trust in yourself.

Seek mentorship: Connect with experienced leaders who can share their wisdom and offer support.

Celebrate small wins: Acknowledge and appreciate your successes, no matter how small they seem. Each positive step reinforces your credibility.

Keep learning: Never stop growing. Read, take courses, ask questions, and seek out new experiences. The more you learn, the more confident you'll become.

Embrace confident action: Confidence often grows with action. Sometimes, you have to step into leadership, even before you feel like a leader. Don't wait for perfect confidence; start acting, and the confidence will follow

Transitioning into leadership is like stepping onto a moving treadmill—you don't get to start at zero, but you can control your pace. The first few months in a management role lay the foundation for long-term success, making it essential to establish credibility, build strong relationships, and refine those all-important problem-solving skills. It's a delicate dance between embracing fresh perspectives and honoring the existing strengths of the team and unit.

One of the quickest ways to gain trust, and it's something often overlooked, is through active listening. Taking the time to truly understand team concerns, workflow challenges, and the nuances of the unit's culture allows you to make informed decisions, rather than imposing change blindly. A fresh perspective is invaluable, absolutely, but leadership is most effective when paired with a genuine awareness of what's already working well. It's about building upon existing strengths, not tearing everything down and starting from scratch.

Quick wins also make a huge difference. Identifying small but meaningful improvements—whether it's streamlining communication channels, adjusting shift assignments to reduce burnout (a critical issue in nursing), or advocating for necessary resources—signals a commitment to both exceptional patient care and staff well-being. These early successes, these tangible improvements, build momentum, foster trust, and boost your own confidence as a leader.

Effective time management becomes a non-negotiable skill. Leadership often comes with a flood of meetings, emails, and administrative tasks. It's easy to get bogged down in the minutiae. But prioritizing staff support and focusing on positive patient outcomes keeps the bigger picture clear. Setting healthy boundaries, delegating effectively (and trusting your team to handle those delegated tasks), and keeping track of long-term strategic goals prevents the role from becoming overwhelming and allows you to focus on the truly important things.

And finally, remember this: leadership isn’t about striving for some unattainable perfection—it’s about adaptability, resilience, and continuous growth. Mistakes will happen; not every decision will be a home run. What sets effective leaders apart isn't their flawless track record, but their ability to learn from missteps, adjust their approach accordingly, and stay engaged in the process. They’re the ones who get back up, dust themselves off, and refine their strategy with each challenge and opportunity.

Now, reflecting on this, consider your own approach to networking. It's a critical component of leadership success. Are there steps you can take, today, to build a more robust and supportive professional network? Think beyond just collecting contacts; focus on cultivating genuine relationships. Who are the individuals whose experience and insights could benefit you? Who are the peers you can support and collaborate with? Building a strong network isn't just about what others can do for you; it's about the mutual support and shared learning that strengthens the entire profession.

CHAPTER 9

LEVERAGING TECHNOLOGY AND INNOVATION

"Technology isn't here to replace us; it's here to help us do our jobs better."
— Unknown

The healthcare landscape has transformed. Gone are the days when a nurse leader's primary concerns were solely staffing, scheduling, and patient needs—addressed through sheer grit and determination. Now, technology has become a force of nature, both a challenge and a powerful solution, fundamentally reshaping decision-making, care delivery, and the very essence of nursing leadership. Imagine a hospital ward where every decision is informed by a wealth of real-time data, where nurses aren't just providing hands-on care but also interpreting complex information, engaging in virtual consultations, and overseeing care across multiple locations. This isn't science fiction; it's the reality of today's nursing, driven largely by the pervasive power of Electronic Health Records (EHRs).

EHRs: A Game-Changer for Decision-Making

EHR systems are like the GPS for healthcare leaders, guiding them through the complexities of patient care. Gone are the days of flipping through paper charts or chasing down test results. But the impact of EHRs goes beyond just convenience. It's about decision-making. In an era when every second counts, having access to a patient's entire health record is priceless.

When a nurse leader needs to make a quick decision — say, adjusting a care plan or ensuring that a medication doesn't interact negatively — they can now rely on a digital tool that provides accurate, up-to-date information. No more relying on memory or outdated notes scribbled on a chart that's been passed around to various care providers. EHRs allow nurse leaders to make data-driven decisions that enhance patient safety and care quality. The result? More effective, efficient leadership.

> *"Technology is nothing. What's important is that you have a faith in people, that they're basically good and smart, and if you give them tools, they'll do wonderful things with them."*
> *— Steve Jobs*

However, as efficient as EHRs are, they're just one piece of the technological puzzle. Data analytics is rapidly becoming the nurse leader's new best friend. Imagine trying to improve patient outcomes or optimize hospital workflows without the ability to interpret trends. You'd be flying blind. But with the power of data analytics, nurse leaders can now track patterns across patient populations, anticipate potential issues, and even predict patient needs before they become problems. This predictive capacity allows healthcare teams to act preemptively rather than reactively — a game-changer when it comes to patient care.

Take patient falls, for instance. A nurse leader with access to data analytics can identify patterns in fall incidents — perhaps a certain time of day, certain medications, or patient demographics — and proactively introduce measures to reduce those incidents. Through analytics, the insights gained don't just help improve operational efficiency but, more importantly, they save lives.

Telehealth is another technology that's opening up new possibilities for nursing leadership. No longer confined to the walls of the hospital or clinic, nursing leadership now extends into the digital realm. Imagine a nurse leader working with patients in remote or underserved communities, guiding them through follow-up care via video calls or helping monitor chronic conditions with mobile apps. With telehealth, a nurse leader's reach goes far beyond the local hospital setting, allowing them to provide consistent care and leadership across vast distances.

It's not just about providing care; it's about creating connections. Telehealth allows for continuous communication with patients, ensuring that follow-ups are more than just a formality. With regular check-ins, nurse leaders can guide their patients toward better health outcomes while simultaneously managing the coordination of care teams across regions.

So, what's the common thread between EHRs, data analytics, and telehealth? Empowerment. These technologies are empowering nurse leaders to step up, make decisions based on real-time data, and provide care that's not only timely but also compassionate. In an era where burnout is a constant concern, these tools give nurse leaders the support they need to manage the complexities of healthcare leadership more effectively.

It's an exciting time to be at the helm of healthcare teams. Technology, though sometimes a bit overwhelming at first, is now a critical enabler of leadership. And as technology continues to evolve, it's safe to say that the role of the nurse leader will only become more dynamic, impactful, and — dare we say — efficient. The key lies in adapting to these tools and embracing the opportunities they offer.

With the right tools, you can do more than just survive — you can thrive. And maybe even squeeze in a coffee break.

In the world of healthcare, time is often the one resource we can't get enough of. For nurse leaders, the demands of overseeing patient care, managing teams, and ensuring everything runs smoothly can feel like juggling flaming torches. The good news? With the right tools, this juggling act doesn't have to be so daunting. Technology has become the ultimate partner for improving workflow and decision-making in nursing leadership, helping streamline processes, enhance communication, and ultimately improve patient care.

Let's start with something that many nurse leaders deal with daily: scheduling and resource management. Balancing staff availability, patient needs, and ensuring that the right resources are in the right place at the right time can feel like a full-time job in itself. Enter scheduling and resource management software. These platforms not only help with shift planning but also allow nurse leaders to track workloads, assess staffing needs, and optimize schedules based on real-time data.

Imagine this: a nurse leader in charge of managing a team of nurses across multiple shifts. Without software, it's easy for things to slip through the cracks — a missed shift change, overworked staff, or a lack of critical supplies. But with resource management software, the nurse leader can plan shifts more efficiently, see where there are gaps in staffing, and even predict potential issues before they arise.

These tools help reduce burnout, ensure adequate staffing, and allow nurse leaders to focus on what matters most — patient care.

Then there's the ever-important aspect of communication. Effective communication is the backbone of successful healthcare leadership. If nurses aren't communicating well with one another, things can quickly spiral out of control. Fortunately, we live in a time when communication is easier than ever. Platforms like Slack, Microsoft Teams, and Zoom (yes, the same one we all know from quarantine life) have become staples in modern healthcare teams. These platforms allow nurse leaders to communicate instantly with their teams, hold virtual meetings, share critical updates, and stay in touch with other departments in real time.

No more waiting for the next shift to pass along vital information. No more relying on scribbled notes passed from one nurse to another. These communication tools have revolutionized how nurse leaders stay connected and collaborate across departments, and the efficiency they bring is undeniable.

But wait, there's more! Predictive analytics is another technology making a huge difference in staffing and patient care management. Nurse leaders have a lot on their plate, and the last thing they need is to be caught off guard by sudden changes in patient volume or an unexpected spike in demand. Predictive analytics uses historical data and trends to anticipate future needs. For example, if data shows that a hospital sees an influx of patients during certain times of the year or after a particular type of surgery, nurse leaders can use that information to staff appropriately, stock supplies, and plan for fluctuations in patient care.

By predicting these changes ahead of time, nurse leaders can avoid chaos and instead respond proactively. It's like having a crystal ball for healthcare management, only much more data-driven and, well, less magical. Predictive analytics helps nurse leaders make decisions that are based on solid evidence rather than guesswork.

And let's not forget about mobile health applications — they've become indispensable for nursing leadership, offering on-the-go access to critical information. Whether it's checking lab results, reviewing a patient's chart, or overseeing care plans, mobile health apps give nurse leaders the freedom to manage patient care and their teams from anywhere. A nurse leader might be on the hospital floor, in a meeting, or even at home when an urgent issue arises. With a mobile app, they can stay on top of things, make quick decisions, and offer guidance in real-time, even when they're not physically present.

One example is MyChart, which allows healthcare providers to access patient records from anywhere, ensuring that nurse leaders are never out of the loop. These apps are also a game-changer when it comes to collaborating with other healthcare professionals, whether they're in the same building or across the country.

In the end, these technological tools don't just make nursing leadership easier; they enhance the overall effectiveness of healthcare teams. They allow nurse leaders to focus on higher-level tasks, like patient advocacy, team building, and strategic planning, while leaving the logistical tasks to the tech. They save time, reduce errors, and, most importantly, help ensure that patient care remains top-notch.

Staying Ahead of Trends and Advocating for Innovation

In healthcare, things move fast. Blink, and suddenly a new technology is revolutionizing patient care, or an emerging trend is reshaping how we think about nursing leadership. As nurse leaders, it's essential not only to keep up with these changes but also to actively advocate for them, ensuring that innovation continues to improve the quality of care we provide. But how do you stay ahead of the curve in an industry that's constantly evolving? And more importantly, how do you convince others that embracing new technologies and practices is the way forward?

First, let's talk about keeping up with emerging healthcare technology. The good news is; you don't have to be a tech wizard to stay informed. There are countless resources out there — from industry blogs and podcasts to conferences and webinars — that can help you keep your finger on the pulse of the latest advancements. But staying updated isn't just about collecting information; it's about filtering it. The key is to focus on the technologies that will genuinely enhance the quality of care, improve operational efficiency, and benefit the teams you lead.

Once you've got your finger on the pulse of innovation, it's time to turn your attention to the people you lead. Encouraging staff adoption of innovative tools is an ongoing challenge for any nurse leader. Change can be intimidating, and it's no surprise that many healthcare professionals are resistant to new technologies or ways of working. As a nurse leader, part of your role is to be the bridge between these advancements and your team. It's about showing them how these tools will make their lives easier, not harder. The goal is to inspire confidence in the technology, not overwhelm them with it.

One way to achieve this is through education. Take the time to show your team how new tools work and why they're beneficial. Lead by example: when your team sees you embracing and utilizing technology, they're more likely to do the same. In one instance, a nurse leader I worked with started implementing a new patient management system. Rather than simply enforcing its use, she took the time to train her team, holding open sessions where they could ask questions, troubleshoot, and share feedback. By making the process collaborative rather than top-down, she ensured that the adoption of the new system wasn't just smooth but embraced by the staff.

It's also important to recognize that some resistance is natural. People don't like change, especially when it's introduced suddenly. As a nurse leader, part of your job is to support your team through the transition. Be patient, listen to their concerns, and address them head-on. Change doesn't happen overnight, but with empathy and strong leadership, it can be successfully managed.

Of course, advocating for innovation isn't just about convincing your team. It's also about championing change at the policy level. Nurse leaders play a crucial role in shaping healthcare policies, especially when it comes to the integration of new technologies and practices. If you believe that a certain innovation could improve patient outcomes or streamline operations, you have a responsibility to advocate for it.

Overcoming resistance to change in healthcare settings often requires more than just convincing your team. It might mean having difficult conversations with administrators or policymakers who are hesitant to invest in new technologies. This is where the power of data comes into play. By presenting solid evidence on how a new tool or process will improve patient care or reduce costs, you can make a compelling case for change. It's not about selling an idea; it's about demonstrating its value.

In my experience, the most successful nurse leaders are those who actively engage with stakeholders, both within and outside their organizations, to ensure that innovation is embraced across all levels. They know that advocacy isn't just about pushing for new technologies — it's about creating a culture that values continuous improvement, whether it's through small updates or major transformations.

As nurse leaders, we have the privilege of shaping the future of healthcare. And while it's not always easy to advocate for change, it's crucial for advancing the care we provide. The future of healthcare isn't about us versus technology; it's about us with technology, building a stronger system together.

The Future of Nursing Leadership and Technology

The future of nursing leadership is no longer a distant concept — it's unfolding right before our eyes, and technology is leading the charge. As we look ahead, we see a landscape where innovations like artificial intelligence, robotics, and virtual reality will play an increasingly vital role in shaping the next generation of nurse leaders. But while these technological advances hold incredible promise, they also come with their own set of challenges and ethical considerations. So, what does the future hold for nursing leadership, and how do we prepare for it?

With great power comes great responsibility. The integration of AI and robotics into nursing will likely raise important questions about the role of human touch in healthcare. After all, while robots may be able to perform certain tasks more efficiently, there's an irreplaceable aspect of nursing that comes from empathy, compassion, and human connection. Nurse leaders will need to balance these new technologies with the human side of care, ensuring that automation enhances, rather than diminishes, the quality of patient experiences.

Virtual reality (VR) is already making waves in nursing education and training. By immersing nurses in realistic virtual environments, VR allows them to practice clinical scenarios, learn new procedures, and refine their skills without the risks associated with traditional training methods. The potential of VR for nursing leadership is vast. As the technology advances, it could revolutionize how nurse leaders train their teams, offering hands-on experience without the constraints of time, resources, or patient safety.

However, the rise of these technologies presents ethical considerations that nursing leaders will need to address. For instance, AI systems rely on vast amounts of data to make predictions, but how do we ensure that this data is accurate, unbiased, and used responsibly? Similarly, while robots may help with routine tasks, they can never replace the compassionate care provided by a nurse. Nurse leaders will have to be the gatekeepers of these technologies, ensuring that they are integrated in a way that enhances patient care while safeguarding the core values of the nursing profession.

The future of nursing leadership isn't just about adapting to new technologies — it's about leading with vision and purpose. Nurse leaders will need to be forward-thinking, constantly looking for opportunities to harness the power of technology to improve healthcare delivery. But at the same time, they must be advocates for the ethical use of these technologies, ensuring that they serve both the healthcare system and the people who rely on it.

Looking even further into the future, robotics may become commonplace in healthcare settings. From surgical robots assisting with complex procedures to robots helping with patient mobility and rehabilitation, nursing leaders will need to stay at the forefront of these advancements. Their role will be to ensure that the integration of robotics into patient care is smooth, beneficial, and most importantly, patient-centered.

And as we look toward these incredible advancements, let's not forget that nursing leadership will always be about people. Yes, technology will continue to play a pivotal role in shaping the healthcare landscape, but it's the nurse leaders who will ultimately determine how these tools are used. The key is not to see technology as a replacement but as an enabler — a way to amplify the already outstanding work that nurses do every day.

As we embrace this technological revolution, let's remember what drives us. Nurse leaders are the ones who guide, support, and inspire their teams. They're the ones who ensure that patient care remains at the heart of everything we do, regardless of the innovations that come our way. After all, the future of nursing leadership is not just about adopting new technologies — it's about harnessing their power to create a more compassionate, efficient, and effective healthcare system.

Taking on a leadership role in nursing can significantly impact your work-life balance, often shifting priorities and increasing demands on your time. To maintain your well-being while growing professionally, it's essential to set clear boundaries between work and personal life, delegate tasks effectively, and prioritize self-care. Leveraging technology, such as scheduling tools and communication platforms, can help streamline tasks, enhance team collaboration, and reduce the time spent on administrative duties, allowing for more focus on patient care and personal time. Ultimately, a sustainable leadership journey requires a balance of professional dedication and personal rejuvenation, ensuring that you lead with clarity, energy, and resilience.

PART 4

LEADING WITH PURPOSE AND VISION

CHAPTER 10

EMPOWERING AND LEADING YOUR TEAM

Think about the best nurse you've ever encountered. What made them stand out? Was it their ability to organize a shift, or was it something more? The words 'manager' and 'leader' are frequently used as synonyms, but in reality, they represent two distinct paths. While both are necessary for a well-functioning team, they require different skill sets and mindsets. If you're a nurse who wants to make a real impact, it's time to understand the crucial difference between being a manager and being a leader.

Managing is primarily concerned with maintaining order, ensuring efficiency, and achieving specific goals through established processes. Managers focus on tasks, resources, and timelines. They are responsible for planning, organizing, directing, and controlling activities to achieve desired outcomes. Think of managing as the operational backbone of a team. A manager ensures the trains run on time, so to speak. They create schedules, delegate tasks, monitor performance, and address any deviations from the plan. They're the ones making sure the budget is balanced, the supplies are ordered, and the paperwork is filed correctly. This is absolutely vital work, and skilled managers are essential.

Leading, on the other hand, is about inspiring, motivating, and empowering individuals to achieve a shared vision. Leaders focus on people, relationships, and creating a culture of growth and development. They don't just tell people *what* to do; they explain *why* it's important and how it contributes to the bigger picture. Leaders are the visionaries, the ones who paint a compelling picture of the future and inspire others to join them on the journey. They build trust, foster collaboration, and create an environment where individuals feel valued, respected, and empowered to reach their full potential. A leader is the conductor of the orchestra, bringing out the best in each individual musician to create a harmonious and impactful symphony.

The key differences can be summarized like this:

Managers: Administer, maintain, focus on systems and processes, rely on control, short-term view, ask "how" and "when," direct people, focus on efficiency.

Leaders: Innovate, develop, focus on people, inspire trust, long-term view, ask "what" and "why," empower people, focus on effectiveness.

In the context of nursing, a manager might be responsible for creating the staffing schedule, ensuring adequate supplies are available, and implementing new protocols. A leader, however, would inspire their team to provide compassionate patient care, advocate for their patients' needs, and continuously seek ways to improve the quality of care. A nurse leader would also foster a culture of learning and professional development within the team, mentoring junior nurses and encouraging them to grow their skills.

It's important to recognize that leadership isn't tied to a specific title or position. You can be a leader regardless of your formal role. A staff nurse can demonstrate leadership by taking initiative, mentoring colleagues, and advocating for patient safety. Leadership is about behavior, not position. It's about the way you interact with others, the influence you have, and the impact you make.

Effective nurse leaders understand that management and leadership are not mutually exclusive. In fact, they are complementary and essential for creating a high-performing team. A successful nurse leader must be able to manage the day-to-day operations of the unit while also inspiring and motivating their team to achieve a shared vision. They must be able to balance the need for efficiency and productivity with the need to support and develop their team members.

Moving from a management mindset to a leadership mindset requires a shift in focus. It requires moving away from simply directing and controlling to empowering and inspiring. It requires cultivating strong interpersonal skills, developing emotional intelligence, and building trusting relationships. It requires a commitment to continuous learning and a genuine desire to help others grow and succeed. It also requires self-awareness. Understanding your own strengths and weaknesses as a leader is crucial for building a strong team and creating a positive work environment. This self-awareness allows you to leverage your strengths and seek support in areas where you may need development. It allows you to recognize your biases and work towards inclusive leadership.

Ultimately, the most effective nurse leaders are those who can seamlessly integrate the skills of management with the qualities of leadership. They are the ones who can not only ensure the smooth operation of their unit but also inspire their team to provide exceptional patient care and make a meaningful difference in the lives of others.

Strategies for Inclusive Leadership and Team Building

Building a high-performing team isn't just about gathering a group of talented individuals; it's about creating an environment where those individuals can thrive, collaborate effectively, and feel a genuine sense of belonging. And in today's diverse healthcare landscape, *inclusive* leadership isn't just a nice-to-have, it's a *must-have*. It's not just ethically right; it's strategically smart. Teams with diverse perspectives make better decisions, are more creative, and are better equipped to serve the diverse patient populations we encounter. This is where the importance of trust, honesty, and consistent support comes into play, as illustrated by this experience: "When building a leadership team, consistency, equality, honesty and truthfulness is the quickest and best way to build trusting relationships. Your team is what makes you successful. They must know and trust that you support them, and you will support them in their independent decisions they make. How you lead and treat your team sets the standard, and you expect them to emulate this as they build their own teams."

Inclusive leadership starts with recognizing that everyone brings unique experiences, backgrounds, and perspectives to the table. It's about not just acknowledging these differences, but actively valuing them and creating a space where everyone feels safe, respected, and empowered to contribute fully. Think of it like planning a potluck dinner. You wouldn't want everyone to bring the *same* dish, would you? Imagine a table groaning under the weight of ten different versions of potato salad. Delicious, perhaps (if you *really* like potato salad), but hardly a diverse and satisfying meal. You'd want a rich and flavorful spread, where each person contributes their favorite recipe, creating a culinary experience that's far more interesting and enjoyable than any single dish could be. That's what inclusive leadership is all about: actively seeking out those diverse 'dishes' – those unique perspectives – and ensuring that everyone has an equal opportunity to share them, creating a richer, more complete, and ultimately, more successful outcome.

So, how do you actually *do* this inclusive leadership thing? Here are a few strategies, building on the foundation of trust highlighted in the anecdote:

Foster Open Communication: Create a culture where team members feel comfortable sharing their ideas, even if they differ from the majority. Encourage active listening and respectful dialogue. Make it clear that disagreements are okay – in fact, they can be a source of innovation – as long as they're expressed constructively. Ask questions like, "What are your thoughts on this?" and "Is there anything we're not considering?" This demonstrates that you value their input. This open communication directly ties into the honesty and truthfulness mentioned in the anecdote. Without open communication, trust cannot be fully established.

Promote Psychological Safety: This is crucial. Team members need to feel safe to take risks, admit mistakes, and ask questions without fear of judgment or reprisal. If people are afraid of being ridiculed or criticized, they'll clam up, and you'll miss out on their valuable contributions. Lead by example – be willing to admit your own mistakes and create a culture where learning from errors is seen as a positive thing (Because everyone makes them. Even you). This ties into the "equality" aspect of the anecdote – everyone should feel equally safe to express themselves.

Embrace Diversity of Thought: Actively seek out different perspectives. Don't just surround yourself with people who agree with you. Challenge your own assumptions and encourage your team to do the same. Invite people with diverse backgrounds, experiences, and skill sets to participate in discussions and decision-making. The more perspectives you have, the better equipped you'll be to tackle complex challenges. This links back to the idea of valuing each team member's unique contribution, as emphasized in the anecdote.

Provide Development Opportunities: Invest in your team's growth and development. Offer mentoring, coaching, and training opportunities to help team members develop their skills and advance their careers. This is especially important for team members from underrepresented groups who may have faced barriers to advancement in the past. By providing equitable access to development opportunities, you're not only helping individuals grow, you're strengthening your entire team. This aligns with the "consistency" mentioned in the anecdote – consistently investing in your team builds trust and demonstrates your commitment to their growth.

Build Trust: Trust, as the anecdote highlights, is the foundation of any strong team. Be transparent, honest, and consistent in your actions. Follow through on your commitments and demonstrate that you genuinely care about your team members' well-being. When your team trusts you, they're more likely to be engaged, motivated, and willing to go the extra mile. This echoes the core message of the anecdote – trust is paramount for team success.

Building an inclusive team takes time, effort, and a genuine commitment to creating a welcoming and supportive environment. It's not something you can just check off a list. It requires ongoing communication, reflection, and a willingness to learn and adapt. But the rewards are well worth the effort. A truly inclusive team, built on a foundation of trust and respect, is a powerful force, capable of achieving remarkable things

Strategies for Motivating and Mentoring Staff

Motivating and mentoring staff are two sides of the same coin. Motivation provides the spark, the initial drive that gets people going. Mentoring provides the fuel, the ongoing support and guidance that keeps them moving forward. As a nurse leader, you need to be skilled at both. It's not enough to simply tell people what to do; you need to inspire them to *want* to do it. And it's not enough to just tell them *how* to do it; you need to guide them, support them, and help them develop their skills so they can do it even better.

Motivation

Motivation is a complex and multifaceted thing. What motivates one person may not motivate another. Some people are driven by financial rewards, while others are more motivated by recognition, autonomy, or a sense of purpose. The key is to understand what drives each individual on your team and tailor your approach accordingly. Here are some strategies for motivating staff:

Recognize and Appreciate Contributions: A little appreciation can go a long way. Publicly acknowledge and celebrate both individual and team accomplishments. A simple "thank you" or a handwritten note can make a big difference. Be specific in your praise. Instead of saying "good job," say "I really appreciate how you handled that difficult patient interaction. Your compassion and professionalism were truly impressive."

Provide Meaningful Work: People are more motivated when they feel that their work has meaning and purpose. Connect their daily tasks to the bigger picture and explain how their contributions make a difference. Help them see how their work impacts patient care and the overall success of the team.

Offer Opportunities for Growth and Development: People are motivated when they feel that they are learning and growing. Provide opportunities for professional development, training, and advancement. Support them in pursuing further education or certifications. Show them that you are invested in their future.

Empower and Delegate: Give team members autonomy and control over their work. Delegate tasks that challenge them and allow them to use their skills. Trust them to make decisions and give them the resources they need to succeed. When people feel empowered, they are more likely to be engaged and motivated.

Create a Positive Work Environment: A positive and supportive work environment can be a powerful motivator. Foster a culture of respect, collaboration, and open communication. Create a space where team members feel valued, appreciated, and supported. A happy team is a productive team.

Set Clear Expectations: Make sure that team members understand what is expected of them. Clearly define their roles, responsibilities, and performance goals. When people know what is expected, they are more likely to be motivated to meet those expectations.

Provide Regular Feedback: Give team members regular feedback on their performance. Be honest and constructive in your feedback. Help them identify areas for improvement and provide them with the support they need to grow. Regular feedback shows that you are paying attention and that you care about their development.

Mentoring

Mentoring is a powerful tool for developing future leaders and fostering a culture of support. It's a one-on-one relationship where an experienced mentor provides guidance, support, and encouragement to a less experienced mentee. Mentoring can help mentees develop their skills, navigate challenges, and achieve their career goals. Here are some tips for effective mentoring:

Build a Strong Relationship: The foundation of any successful mentoring relationship is trust and rapport. Get to know your mentee on a personal level. Show genuine interest in their career goals and aspirations.

Provide Guidance and Support: Offer your mentee advice, guidance, and support. Share your own experiences and insights. Help them navigate challenges and make informed decisions.

Be a Role Model: Be the kind of leader you want your mentee to become. Demonstrate the qualities and behaviors you want them to emulate.

Encourage Self-Reflection: Help your mentee reflect on their strengths, weaknesses, and goals. Ask open-ended questions that encourage them to think critically about their own development.

Offer Constructive Feedback: Provide your mentee with honest and constructive feedback. Help them identify areas for improvement and provide them with the support they need to grow.

Be Patient and Supportive: Mentoring is a long-term commitment. Be patient and supportive. Celebrate your mentee's successes and help them through their challenges.

Motivating and mentoring staff are essential skills for any nurse leader. By creating a positive and supportive work environment, recognizing contributions, offering growth opportunities, and providing guidance and support, you can empower your team to achieve extraordinary things. It's about investing in your people, helping them grow, and inspiring them to reach their full potential. And when your team succeeds, you succeed.

So, as you navigate your own leadership journey, remember this: setbacks are inevitable, but resilience is a choice. Reflect on your own experiences with adversity. What lessons have you learned? How have those challenges shaped the leader you are today? Because true leadership, as Bill Bradley so wisely stated, is about 'unlocking people's potential to become better.' And that includes unlocking our *own* potential to learn, grow, and bounce back. By embracing resilience, not just for ourselves but for our teams, we create a culture where everyone can thrive, learn from their mistakes, and ultimately, become the best versions of themselves. It's in those moments of challenge, when we rise again, that we truly discover the power of leadership – and the potential within ourselves and those we lead.

CHAPTER 11

ADVOCACY AND INFLUENCE

Advocacy is a cornerstone of effective nursing leadership. It's about using your voice and influence to champion the needs of your patients, your team, and the nursing profession as a whole. While advocating for individual patients is a fundamental aspect of nursing practice, nurse leaders must also be skilled at advocating for nurses themselves, particularly at the organizational level. This means working to improve working conditions, ensure adequate resources, promote professional development, and create a culture where nurses feel valued and supported. It's about ensuring that nurses have the tools and the environment they need to provide the best possible care.

Advocating for nurses at the organizational level requires a multifaceted approach. It's not just about raising concerns; it's about proposing solutions, building coalitions, and influencing decision-making processes. It requires strong communication skills, political savvy, and the ability to build relationships with key stakeholders. It also requires a deep understanding of the organizational structure, policies, and power dynamics. For you to be able to effectively advocate for nurses within your organization, you'll need good strategies.

Understand the Organizational Landscape: Before you can effectively advocate for change, you need to understand how your organization works. Identify the key decision-makers, understand the organizational culture, and learn how policies are developed and implemented. Who has the power to make the changes you're seeking? What are their priorities? Understanding the organizational landscape will help you tailor your approach and increase your chances of success.

Build Relationships: Relationships are essential for effective advocacy. Build strong relationships with key stakeholders, including other nurses, physicians, administrators, and members of the leadership team. The stronger your relationships, the more likely people will be to listen to your concerns and consider your proposals. Networking is essential here. Attend meetings, join committees, and participate in organizational initiatives. Get to know the people who can help you make a difference.

Gather Data and Evidence: Effective advocacy is based on data and evidence. Don't just rely on anecdotal evidence. Gather data to support your claims and demonstrate the need for change. For example, if you're advocating for improved staffing ratios, collect data on patient outcomes, nurse satisfaction, and staff turnover. The more data you have, the more persuasive your arguments will be.

Frame Your Arguments Effectively: How you frame your arguments can make a big difference. Focus on the benefits of the changes you're proposing, not just the problems. Explain how the changes will improve patient care, enhance staff satisfaction, or reduce costs. Frame your arguments in a way that resonates with the decision-makers you're trying to influence. For instance, instead of focusing on how understaffing creates stress for nurses, frame it as how adequate staffing improves patient safety, reduces readmissions, and improves the hospital's overall quality rating.

Propose Solutions, Not Just Problems: Don't just complain about problems. Propose solutions. When you present a problem, be prepared to offer concrete suggestions for how it can be addressed. This demonstrates that you're not just a complainer, but a problem-solver. It also increases the likelihood that your proposals will be taken seriously.

Build Coalitions: You're more likely to be successful if you have the support of others. Build coalitions with other nurses, physicians, and other stakeholders who share your concerns. The more people you have on your side; the more influence you'll have. Strength in numbers matters.

Be Persistent and Patient: Change doesn't happen overnight. Advocacy requires persistence and patience. Don't get discouraged if your initial efforts are unsuccessful. Keep advocating for your cause and don't give up. Sometimes, it takes time for people to be persuaded. Be willing to try different approaches and be open to compromise.

Know Your Rights: Understand your rights as a nurse and the legal and regulatory framework that governs nursing practice. This will empower you to advocate for yourself and your colleagues effectively. If your organization is violating regulations or infringing on nurses' rights, you need to know how to address the situation.

Use Your Voice: Don't be afraid to speak up. Your voice matters. Nurses are trusted professionals, and your opinions are valued. Use your voice to advocate for your patients, your team, and your profession. The more nurses who speak up, the more likely we are to make a difference.

Advocating for nurses at the organizational level is about creating a work environment, where nurses are empowered to provide the best possible care and where their voices are heard and respected. By using the strategies outlined above, nurse leaders can become effective advocates for their teams and contribute to positive change within their organizations.

While advocating for nurses is essential, sometimes the most impactful changes come from influencing the very policies and organizational culture that shape their work environment. This section focuses on the *how* – the specific strategies and tactics nurse leaders can use to navigate the complexities of organizational change and create a more supportive and effective system for nurses.

Influencing policy and culture is about more than just having good ideas; it's about understanding how to navigate the system to bring those ideas to fruition. It requires a deep understanding of organizational dynamics, political savvy, and the ability to build consensus and momentum. It's about understanding where the levers of power lie and how to use them effectively to influence policy changes and organizational culture.

Map the Power Dynamics: Before you embark on a policy change initiative, take the time to map out the power dynamics within your organization. Identify the key decision-makers, understand their priorities, and assess their influence. Who are the formal and informal leaders? Who holds the purse strings? Who are the key influencers? Understanding the power structure will help you identify the most effective channels for influencing change.

Build Relationships Strategically: Don't just build relationships with people you like; build relationships with people who can help you achieve your goals. Identify the individuals who have the power to make the changes you're seeking and cultivate relationships with them. This might involve attending meetings, joining committees, or simply having informal conversations. Focus on building genuine connections based on mutual respect and shared goals.

Frame Your Message for the Audience: Different people are motivated by different things. When you're advocating for a policy change, tailor your message to the specific audience you're trying to reach. What are their priorities? What are their concerns? How can you frame your proposal in a way that resonates with them? For example, if you're trying to persuade the CFO, focus on the financial benefits of the change. If you're trying to persuade frontline nurses, focus on how the change will improve their working conditions.

Use Data and Storytelling: Data is essential for making a compelling case, but data alone isn't always enough. Combine data with storytelling to make your message more memorable and impactful. Share real-life examples of how the current policy is affecting nurses and patients. Use stories to illustrate the benefits of the proposed change. Data provides the facts, but stories provide the emotional connection.

Find Allies and Build Coalitions: Change is rarely achieved alone. Identify individuals and groups who share your concerns and build coalitions with them. The more voices you have supporting your cause, the more likely you are to be heard. Look for allies within and outside of your department. Don't be afraid to reach out to other organizations or professional associations for support.

Pilot Test and Refine: Before implementing a policy change organization-wide, consider pilot testing it in a smaller setting. This allows you to gather data on the effectiveness of the change and make any necessary adjustments before rolling it out more broadly. A successful pilot test can be a powerful tool for persuading others to adopt the change.

Be Patient and Persistent: Changing policy and organizational culture is a marathon, not a sprint. It takes time, effort, and persistence. Don't get discouraged if your initial efforts are met with resistance. Keep advocating for your cause and be patient. Sometimes, the most significant changes take years to achieve.

Celebrate Successes and Learn from Failures: When you achieve a policy change, celebrate your success! Acknowledge the contributions of everyone who helped make it happen. This will motivate others to get involved in future initiatives. And when you encounter setbacks, don't be afraid to learn from your failures. Analyze what went wrong and use those lessons to improve your approach next time.

Real advocacy isn't confined to patient rooms or community outreach; it extends to the very heart of decision-making. Effective nurse leaders understand this, recognizing that their voices must be heard where policies are forged and organizational strategies are shaped. It's about more than just having a seat at the table; it's about actively participating, bringing the unique insights and frontline experiences of nurses to the forefront.

Imagine a hospital-wide meeting buzzing with talk of a new electronic health record (EHR) system. A nurse leader, rather than passively observing, seizes the opportunity. They don't just ask *if* nurses were consulted; they drill down on *how* that feedback was incorporated. They don't simply point out potential problems; they offer concrete solutions, drawing on their team's on-the-ground experience to suggest modifications to the EHR interface that could prevent patient safety risks and alleviate the already heavy workload of nurses. This isn't just about voicing concerns; it's about shaping the conversation, influencing decisions, and ultimately, ensuring that the EHR implementation serves both patients and the nurses who care for them. *That's* the power of nurse leadership in action

Activity (Yes, Get Your Journal Out)

Think about a time you advocated for something, whether it was a small change on your unit or a larger initiative within your organization. What strategies did you use? What were the challenges you faced? What were the outcomes?

Now, consider a different scenario: You want to advocate for a change in your organization's policy regarding mandatory overtime. Nurses on your unit are experiencing burnout due to excessive overtime, and you believe it's impacting patient care.

Activity:

Map the Landscape: Who are the key decision-makers regarding this policy? Who are the potential allies? Who might be resistant to change?

Gather Your Evidence: What data can you collect to support your case? Consider things like overtime hours logged, staff turnover rates, patient satisfaction scores, and even anecdotal stories from nurses about how mandatory overtime is affecting them.

Craft Your Message: How will you frame your argument? Will you focus on the impact on patient safety? The financial costs of burnout and turnover? The ethical implications of forcing nurses to work excessive hours? Tailor your message to resonate with your audience (e.g., the CFO, the CNO, the HR director).

Practice Your Pitch: Imagine you're presenting your case to the hospital's policy committee. Practice articulating your points clearly and persuasively. Anticipate potential questions or objections and prepare your responses.

Build Your Coalition: Who are the other nurses or stakeholders who might support your cause? Reach out to them and ask for their help. A strong coalition can amplify your voice and increase your chances of success.

This activity encourages you to apply the concepts discussed in the chapter to a real-world scenario. By mapping the landscape, gathering evidence, crafting your message, practicing your pitch, and building a coalition, you can develop a comprehensive strategy for advocating for change and representing the voice of nurses in decision-making rooms. This kind of practical application reinforces the learning and prepares you to be a more effective advocate in your own professional practice.

CHAPTER 12

MAINTAINING BALANCE AND AVOIDING BURNOUT

Nurse leaders are often so busy caring for others – their patients, their teams, their organizations – that they forget to care for themselves. This is a recipe for burnout, a state of emotional, physical, and mental exhaustion brought on by prolonged or repeated stress. And a burned-out leader is not an effective leader. Prioritizing well-being and setting boundaries isn't selfish; it's essential for sustainable leadership. It's about recognizing that you can't pour from an empty cup. As this anecdote illustrates, neglecting self-care can have significant consequences: "Not all managers are "good" managers or managers you want to emulate. However, you can learn so much from these leaders and NOT WHAT TO DO. My first director had truly adopted the laissez-faire managerial style. He never met with me, except for my yearly evaluation and I rarely saw him on the unit. However, of all the leaders I've had, I learned the most from him….and what NOT to DO, and how not to treat my staff, etc.

The only positive thing I can say about laissez-faire leaders, is the amount of autonomy you have. I basically acted as the manager and director of my unit and made high-level decisions. In hindsight, I probably should not have been making. However, if the unit ran smoothly and no one was complaining to senior leadership, I had free reign. Unfortunately, one of the most frustrating aspects of a laissez-faire leader is their lack of care for you and the unit. When I as the manager and had exhausted all my resources to solve an issue/problem, and I needed "director" approval or input…..his typically response was to shrug his shoulders and asked "why are you asking me"? This leader ultimately was the reason I left this managerial role due to burnout, lack of authority and inability to be a change-agent, etc." This leader's neglect not only impacted their team but likely contributed to their own burnout, demonstrating the interconnectedness of leadership and self-care.

Self-care isn't just about bubble baths and massages (though those can be nice too!). It's about implementing practical strategies that address the specific demands of nurse leadership. It's about creating a sustainable rhythm that allows you to thrive, not just survive. Here are some tailored self-care strategies for nurse leaders:

Schedule "Me Time": This sounds simple, but it's often the first thing to go. Treat appointments with yourself just as you would any other important meeting. Block out time in your calendar for activities you enjoy, whether it's reading, exercising, spending time with loved ones, or simply doing nothing. Protect this time fiercely. It's not a luxury; it's a necessity.

Set Boundaries: Nurse leaders are often bombarded with requests and demands. It's essential to set boundaries to protect your time and energy. Learn to say "no" gracefully but firmly. Delegate tasks when possible. Don't be afraid to disconnect from work outside of designated hours. Establish clear expectations about your availability and stick to them.

Prioritize Sleep: Sleep deprivation is a major contributor to burnout. Aim for 7-8 hours of quality sleep each night. Create a relaxing bedtime routine and make sure your bedroom is conducive to sleep. Avoid caffeine and alcohol before bed. If you're struggling with sleep, talk to your doctor.

Nourish Your Body: Eat a healthy diet and stay hydrated. Fuel your body with nutritious foods that will give you the energy you need to handle the demands of your job. Limit processed foods, sugary drinks, and excessive caffeine.

Move Your Body: Exercise is a powerful stress reliever. Find an activity you enjoy and make it a regular part of your routine. Even a short walk during your lunch break can make a difference. Physical activity not only improves your physical health but also boosts your mood and reduces stress.

Practice Mindfulness: Mindfulness techniques, such as meditation or deep breathing exercises, can help you manage stress and stay grounded in the present moment. Even a few minutes of mindfulness each day can make a difference. There are many apps and resources available to help you get started.

Connect with Others: Social connection is essential for well-being. Spend time with loved ones, connect with colleagues, and build a strong support network. Talking about your challenges and sharing your experiences can be incredibly helpful.

Seek Support: Don't be afraid to ask for help when you need it. Talk to a trusted friend, family member, or therapist. Consider joining a support group for nurse leaders. Seeking support is a sign of strength, not weakness.

Reassess Your Workload: If you're consistently feeling overwhelmed, it's time to reassess your workload. Are there tasks you can delegate? Are there projects you can postpone? Are you taking on too much? Don't be afraid to ask for help from your supervisor or colleagues.

Find Joy and Meaning: Remember why you became a nurse leader in the first place. Reconnect with your passion for nursing and find joy in your work. Celebrate your accomplishments and focus on the positive impact you're making.

Self-care is not a one-size-fits-all approach. What works for one person may not work for another. Experiment with different strategies and find what works best for you. The key is to make self-care a priority and integrate it into your daily life. It's an investment in yourself, your team, and your leadership.

Recognizing Signs of Burnout and Addressing Them Proactively

Burnout isn't something that happens overnight. It's a gradual process, a slow erosion of your emotional, physical, and mental reserves. Recognizing the signs early is crucial for preventing it from becoming overwhelming and debilitating. Ignoring the warning signs can lead to serious consequences, not just for your own well-being, but for your team and your patients. A burned-out leader is less effective, less compassionate, and more prone to errors.

Burnout manifests in various ways, impacting different people differently. It's essential to be aware of the common signs and symptoms, both in yourself and in your team members. These can be categorized into:

Emotional Exhaustion: This is the feeling of being emotionally drained and depleted. You may feel irritable, cynical, or detached. You might have a short fuse and react strongly to minor stressors.

You may also experience a decreased sense of personal accomplishment, feeling like no matter how hard you try, it's never enough.

Physical Exhaustion: This is the feeling of being physically tired and run down. You may experience fatigue, insomnia, headaches, muscle aches, or other physical symptoms. You might find it difficult to concentrate or focus. Your immune system may be weakened, making you more susceptible to illness.

Cognitive Exhaustion: This involves difficulties with concentration, memory, and decision-making. You might feel overwhelmed by even simple tasks. You may struggle to think clearly or creatively. You may also experience a sense of detachment or depersonalization, feeling like you're going through the motions without really being present.

Recognizing Burnout in Yourself

Are you constantly feeling tired, even after a good night's sleep?

Do you find yourself becoming easily irritated or frustrated with your team or patients?

Have you lost interest in activities you used to enjoy?

Are you struggling to concentrate or make decisions?

Do you feel like you're just going through the motions at work?

Are you experiencing physical symptoms like headaches, muscle aches, or sleep problems?

Are you isolating yourself from friends, family, or colleagues?

Do you dread going to work?

Recognizing Burnout in Others

Increased absenteeism or tardiness

Decreased productivity or performance

Changes in mood or behavior (e.g., irritability, cynicism, withdrawal)

Complaints of fatigue or physical symptoms

Difficulty concentrating or making decisions

Negative or pessimistic attitude

Lack of engagement or enthusiasm

Increased errors or near misses

The key to addressing burnout is to take action *before* it becomes severe. Early intervention is crucial. Here are some proactive steps you can take:

Self-Assessment: Regularly check in with yourself and assess your own well-being. Be honest about how you're feeling and don't dismiss the warning signs.

Open Communication: Talk to your supervisor, colleagues, or a trusted mentor about how you're feeling. Don't be afraid to ask for help. Sharing your concerns can be a cathartic experience and can lead to practical solutions.

Seek Professional Help: If you're experiencing significant symptoms of burnout, don't hesitate to seek professional help. A therapist or counselor can provide support and guidance.

Implement Self-Care Strategies: Prioritize the self-care strategies discussed in the previous section. Make sure you're getting enough sleep, eating a healthy diet, exercising regularly, and engaging in activities you enjoy.

Set Boundaries and Delegate: Learn to say "no" to requests that will overload you. Delegate tasks when possible and don't be afraid to ask for help.

Reassess Your Workload: If you're consistently feeling overwhelmed, talk to your supervisor about adjusting your workload. It's important to have a manageable workload that allows you to maintain a healthy work-life balance.

Take Breaks: Regular breaks are essential for preventing burnout. Take short breaks throughout the day to recharge your batteries. Use your vacation time to disconnect from work and relax.

Create a Supportive Work Environment: As a leader, you play a crucial role in creating a supportive work environment for your team. Encourage open communication, promote work-life balance, and recognize and appreciate their contributions. Be mindful of the workload you assign to your team members and be willing to offer support when needed.

Addressing burnout is an ongoing process, not a one-time fix. It requires a commitment to self-care, open communication, and a willingness to make changes. By recognizing the signs early and taking proactive steps, you can prevent burnout from taking hold and maintain a healthy and fulfilling leadership career.

Finding Fulfillment and Longevity in a Leadership Career

Nurse leadership is more than a job; it's a calling, a chance to shape the future of healthcare. But the path isn't always smooth. The daily grind can dim even the brightest passion. Finding true fulfillment and building a lasting career isn't about just surviving the challenges; it's about thriving amidst them. It's about keeping that inner fire burning and finding real meaning in your work.

What ignites one leader might not spark another. Fulfillment is a deeply personal quest. But there are common threads that weave through the stories of those who find true joy in leading. It starts with remembering why you chose this path. What drew you to nursing? What inspired you to lead? Reconnecting with those core values, that initial "why," can reignite a flickering flame. Think back to those moments in your career that truly resonated. What made them special? How can you create more of those experiences?

True fulfillment often comes from making a tangible difference. As a nurse leader, you have the power to touch lives – patients, your team, the entire healthcare system. Focus on those moments when your leadership truly mattered. Did you advocate for a patient and see a positive outcome? Did you mentor a junior nurse and watch them blossom? Celebrating these wins, big and small, reinforces your sense of purpose.

The healthcare world never stands still. So, neither can you. Lifelong learning isn't just a good idea; it's essential for staying engaged and inspired. Embrace new knowledge, seek out fresh perspectives, and never stop growing. Conferences, journals, mentors – use them all to fuel your intellectual curiosity. A stagnant leader risks burnout, pure and simple.

Sharing your expertise with others is another powerful source of fulfillment. Mentoring aspiring leaders isn't just about giving back; it's about solidifying your own understanding and appreciation of your craft. Guiding others can reignite your own passion in unexpected ways.

Strong connections are vital. Nurture relationships with your team, your colleagues, and other leaders. Build a network of support that understands the unique challenges you face. Sharing experiences, offering advice, and simply knowing you're not alone can make all the difference.

And let's be real: balance matters. It's not just about self-care (though that's crucial too). It's about creating a life where work and personal joy coexist. Make time for the things that recharge you – family, hobbies, relaxation. A well-rounded leader is a more effective leader.

Change is inevitable, especially in healthcare. Don't resist it; embrace it. See change as a chance to grow, to innovate, to lead in new and exciting ways. A flexible mindset is your best defense against career stagnation.

Set goals. What do you want to achieve as a leader? What kind of impact do you want to make? Break those big dreams into smaller, manageable steps. Celebrate each milestone along the way. It's a journey, after all.

Explore your passions. What area of nurse leadership truly excites you? Patient safety? Leadership development? Finding your niche can help you focus your energy and make a more profound contribution.

Striving to leave a meaningful mark on the profession can provide a deep sense of purpose that sustains you through the ups and downs of leadership. This journey of finding fulfillment and building a lasting career is a marathon, not a sprint. It demands self-reflection, a commitment to growth, and a genuine desire to make a difference. By nurturing your "why," embracing continuous learning, building strong connections, and finding balance, you can create a leadership career that is both fulfilling and enduring.

Finding fulfillment and longevity in leadership often means having a real impact, and that impact frequently comes from having a voice in the rooms where decisions are made. It's not enough to simply *have* a seat at the table; you need to know how to use your voice effectively. This isn't about grandstanding or self-promotion; it's about strategically representing the needs and perspectives of your fellow nurses. It's about bringing the realities of frontline nursing to the forefront of policy discussions and resource allocation. It's about ensuring that the voices of those who provide direct patient care are heard and valued by those who make the big decisions.

Consider this: A hospital committee is debating the implementation of a new staffing model. A nurse leader, present in that meeting, doesn't just passively listen. They actively engage, asking pointed questions about how the proposed model will impact workload, patient safety, and nurse satisfaction. They share concrete examples from their unit, illustrating the potential challenges and unintended consequences of the new system. They don't just point out the problems; they offer alternative solutions, drawing on their team's experience and expertise.

They understand that their role is not just to represent their own opinions, but to amplify the collective voice of the nurses they lead. By bringing this frontline perspective to the table, they can influence the decision-making process and ensure that the final outcome is one that truly benefits both nurses and patients. This is how nurse leaders translate their passion for their profession into tangible change.

Think about your leadership legacy. What do you want to be remembered for as a nurse leader, and how can you work toward that vision now? Imagine it's ten years from now, and a colleague is describing your contributions to nursing. What stories would they tell? What impact would you have made? Consider not just your professional achievements, but also the kind of leader you were – your compassion, your integrity, your dedication to your team. What steps can you take *today* to start building that legacy? Perhaps it's mentoring a junior nurse, advocating for a policy change, or simply making a conscious effort to lead with kindness and empathy. Your legacy isn't something you create at the end of your career; it's something you build day by day, through every interaction, every decision, and every act of leadership.

> *"Almost everything will work again if you unplug it for a few minutes, including you."*
>
> **– Anne Lamott**

This quote serves as a powerful reminder that self-care isn't a weakness; it's a necessity, especially for leaders who are constantly giving of themselves. Just like any machine, we need time to unplug, recharge, and reconnect with ourselves. Prioritizing our well-being is not selfish; it's an essential part of being an effective leader. Only when we care for ourselves can we truly care for others and lead with compassion, strength, and resilience.

PART 5

MEN IN NURSING AND LEADERSHIP OPPORTUNITIES

CHAPTER 13

BREAKING BARRIERS AND CHALLENGING STEREOTYPES

Once upon a time, in a world where pink was synonymous with nurturing and blue represented strength, nursing became inextricably linked to the feminine. It wasn't always this way; historical records reveal a more nuanced picture. However, over centuries, societal norms, deeply ingrained stereotypes, and the evolving structure of healthcare itself shaped a narrative that cast nursing as primarily a woman's domain.

In its early days, nursing, while considered a noble and compassionate profession, was often less a chosen career path and more an extension of perceived female domestic roles. The caregiving inherent in nursing was seen as a natural outgrowth of women's supposed innate nurturing abilities. Religious orders frequently established and ran hospitals, further solidifying this connection, as nursing became a vocation for women who saw it as a spiritual calling. The image of the "angel of the house," clad in a pristine white apron and starched cap, emerged as the quintessential representation of the nurse—a figure defined by unwavering dedication to care, compassion, and selflessness. This idealized image, while celebrating the virtues of caregiving, also inadvertently reinforced the gendered nature of the profession.

But what about the men? Their presence in nursing, though less visible, was nonetheless significant. Historically, men in nursing were often relegated to specific niches, most notably within military contexts. They cared for wounded soldiers on the battlefield, providing essential medical attention amidst the chaos of war. Yet, even in these roles, their contributions were frequently overshadowed by the larger narrative of war heroism. The softer, more romanticized portrayal of female caregivers further marginalized the contributions of male nurses. Their stories, their dedication, and their skills were often relegated to the background, lost in the broader historical narrative.

As the 20th century dawned, the world underwent significant social and cultural shifts. Yet, despite these changes, the stereotype of nursing as a female profession persisted. Men remained largely absent from civilian nursing roles, facing both societal biases and institutional barriers. The profession, even as it professionalized and expanded, remained stubbornly dominated by women, perpetuating the idea that caring for the sick and vulnerable was inherently a feminine trait. This historical context is crucial to understanding the present-day realities of gender in nursing and the ongoing efforts to create a more inclusive and representative profession.

Stereotypes are funny things. They're like invisible walls that keep people out, no matter how capable they are. And for men in nursing, those walls were particularly tall.

The bias against men in nursing is rooted in deeply ingrained societal expectations. From a young age, boys are often encouraged to pursue careers in fields like engineering, medicine, or business—anything that requires strength, intellect, or leadership. Nursing, with its focus on compassion and care, was rarely seen as a masculine pursuit. Even today, the image of a nurse is often that of a woman, perpetuating the idea that nursing is "women's work."

But here's the thing: nursing isn't just about caregiving; it's about science, technology, and leadership. It's about saving lives, managing crises, and making tough decisions. These are skills that don't belong to any particular gender. Yet, the stigma persists.

The Impact on Men: A Battle Against Expectations

Imagine trying to build a house when everyone keeps telling you that only women can hammer nails. That's what it feels like for many men who choose nursing as a career.

The underrepresentation of men in nursing has real consequences. For one, it limits the pool of talent available to the profession. With nearly 90% of nurses being women, the perspectives and experiences that men could bring to the table are often overlooked. But it's not just about numbers—it's about the unique contributions men can make.

Men in nursing often face skepticism, whether from patients, colleagues, or even themselves. They may question whether they fit in, whether they're "man enough" for the job. This internal struggle can be exhausting, especially when society continues to reinforce outdated stereotypes.

But here's the kicker: men who do choose nursing aren't just changing the profession—they're challenging the very notion of what it means to be a caregiver. And that's a powerful thing. While the road has been long, there are signs that things are changing. More men are stepping into nursing, and they're making a difference.

Over the past few decades, the number of male nurses has slowly but steadily increased. While still a minority, they are becoming more visible and respected within the profession. Many of these men are not only nurses but also leaders—men like you, who have broken through the glass ceiling and are now paving the way for others.

These trailblazers are not just fighting for their own place in the profession; they're advocating for change. They're showing that nursing is not a gender-specific role but a profession that thrives on diversity and inclusivity. By doing so, they're helping to dismantle the stereotypes that have held men back for so long.

And let's be honest—when a man walks into a hospital room, people notice. Not because he's a nurse, but because he's a man in a traditionally female-dominated field. That attention can be both a blessing and a curse, but it's also an opportunity to challenge assumptions and open minds.

How Men Bring Unique Perspectives to Nursing Leadership

Imagine walking into a room filled with mirrors. Each mirror reflects something different—some show you in a suit, others in scrubs, and a few even in superhero capes. That's what it's like for men in nursing leadership—each one reflects a unique combination of skills, experiences, and perspectives.

Men in nursing leadership bring a distinct set of strengths and perspectives that complement the skills of their female counterparts. These differences aren't about being better or worse; they're about adding layers to the tapestry of leadership. Here's why men matter in nursing leadership:

•Problem-Solving Approaches: Men often approach problem-solving with a focus on strategy and systems thinking. They excel at analyzing complex situations and devising practical solutions. Think of it like playing chess—men in leadership tend to look several moves ahead, anticipating potential challenges and crafting plans to mitigate them. This can be particularly valuable in high-pressure environments like emergency rooms or intensive care units.

•Communication Styles: While many men are stereotyped as less empathetic, the truth is that men can bring a different kind of communication style—one that is often more direct and solution-focused. Picture a nurse who doesn't just listen but also knows when to say, "Let's get this done." This can be incredibly effective in crisis management, where clear, concise communication is crucial.

•Leadership Philosophies: Men in leadership often bring a sense of accountability and responsibility that can be refreshing in a field traditionally dominated by women. They tend to prioritize fairness, transparency, and a structured approach to decision-making, which can help create a more balanced leadership environment. It's like having a GPS in a world of maps—clear directions and a steady hand.

Collaboration is like a dance—when everyone moves in harmony, magic happens. But when you mix in different rhythms and styles, the dance becomes even more captivating. Diverse leadership teams, including men, enhance collaboration in several ways:

- **Broader Perspectives:** A team with varied backgrounds and experiences can tackle challenges from multiple angles. This diversity of thought leads to more creative and effective solutions. Imagine a leadership team where every member brings a unique perspective—whether it's from military service, corporate management, or grassroots community work. The result? A more well-rounded approach to patient care and organizational strategy.

- **Improved Decision-Making:** Studies show that diverse teams make better decisions. When leaders come from different walks of life, they bring a wider range of knowledge and experiences. This leads to more informed and thoughtful decision-making, which is critical in healthcare settings. It's like having a panel of experts instead of just one opinion—more voices, more wisdom.

•Enhanced Innovation: Innovation thrives in environments where people challenge each other's assumptions. A diverse team encourages fresh ideas and out-of-the-box thinking, leading to breakthroughs in patient care, operational efficiency, and staff engagement. It's like mixing ingredients in a recipe—you never know what delicious dish you'll end up with.

Real-World Examples: How Men Are Making a Difference

Real-life stories often best illustrate a point, and the history of nursing offers compelling examples of men who have not only thrived in leadership roles but also significantly shaped the profession. From ancient temple priests to battlefield combat medics, men have a long, though often overlooked, history in nursing. Despite societal shifts that gradually feminized the field, their contributions persisted, paving the way for the increasing number of male nurses today. These trailblazers challenged traditional norms, broke down barriers, and ultimately enriched the profession with their diverse skills and perspectives.

James Derham's story is one of extraordinary resilience. Born into slavery, he learned medicine from his owners, becoming the first African American formally recognized as a medical practitioner in the U.S. His post-freedom practice exemplified his dedication to healing, a powerful testament to the human spirit's ability to overcome adversity.

Walt Whitman, the famed poet, traded his pen for a nurse's uniform during the Civil War. Caring for wounded soldiers profoundly impacted him, inspiring his poignant poem "The Wound Dresser." Whitman's experience highlights the emotional and spiritual dimensions of nursing, reminding us of the power of human connection in healing.

LeRoy Craig was a champion for both male nurses and fair compensation. He successfully advocated for the Bolton Act, granting men equal status in the military nurse corps. Recognizing that fair wages are essential to attracting and retaining talent, he also fought for increased pay for nurses, benefiting both men and women in the profession.

Edward T. Lyon shattered barriers in military nursing. He became the first man commissioned as a reserve officer in the U.S. Nurse Corps, opening doors for men to serve in professional nursing roles within the armed forces. His leadership paved the way for greater inclusion and recognition of male nurses in the military.

Joe Hogan's fight for educational access reached the Supreme Court. Denied admission to a women-only nursing school, he challenged the discriminatory practice, ultimately winning the right to pursue his bachelor's degree. His case, Mississippi University for Women v. Hogan, was a landmark victory for gender equality in nursing education.

These men, and countless others, represent the diverse paths to nursing leadership. Their stories underscore the importance of perseverance, advocacy, and the enduring contributions of men to a profession that benefits from the skills and perspectives of all.

The Ripple Effect: How Men in Leadership Impact the Profession

When men step into leadership roles in nursing, they don't just change their own careers—they ripple through the entire profession.

Inspiring Future Generations: Men in leadership roles serve as role models for younger generations, challenging the notion that nursing is a "woman's profession." Their success stories can inspire other men to consider nursing as a viable and rewarding career path. After all, if men can lead hospitals and manage critical care units, why can't they be nurses too?

Breaking Down Barriers: By demonstrating that men can excel in nursing leadership, these trailblazers help break down the barriers that have historically kept men out of the profession. They pave the way for greater acceptance and open doors for future generations of male nurses. It's like knocking down a wall that was built on a faulty foundation—once it falls, everyone benefits.

Driving Change in Policy and Practice: Men in leadership positions often advocate for changes that benefit the entire profession. They push for policies that address burnout, improve work-life balance, and ensure that nurses are valued for their expertise. Their influence extends beyond their immediate teams, shaping the future of healthcare delivery. It's like planting seeds that grow into trees—small actions today lead to big changes tomorrow.

Enhancing Patient Care: Ultimately, the impact of men in leadership roles is felt most profoundly in patient care. A diverse leadership team brings a wider range of experiences and perspectives, leading to more innovative and effective care practices. Patients benefit from this enhanced care, and the entire healthcare system becomes stronger and more resilient. It's like adding spices to a dish—each one enhances the flavor, making the whole meal more satisfying.

Men in nursing leadership bring a unique set of strengths and perspectives that enrich the profession. From problem-solving and communication to innovation and inspiration, their contributions are invaluable. By embracing diversity in leadership, we create a more dynamic, effective, and compassionate healthcare system.

So, the next time someone asks why men should be in nursing leadership, you can smile and say, 'Because a symphony needs more than just violins.'

> *Diversity is not about how we differ; it's about embracing one another's uniqueness.*
> *– Ola Joseph*

Embracing Diversity in Leadership

Embracing diversity in leadership is not just a nice-to-have—it's essential for the success of any organization. A diverse leadership team brings together a wide range of perspectives, experiences, and talents, leading to better decision-making, innovation, and ultimately, better patient care.

Better Decision-Making: Diverse teams consider a broader range of options and perspectives, leading to more informed and effective decisions. This is especially crucial in healthcare, where quick and accurate decisions can mean the difference between life and death.

Innovation and Creativity: Different backgrounds and experiences fuel creativity and innovation. A diverse team is more likely to come up with groundbreaking solutions to complex problems, driving progress in patient care and healthcare delivery.

Stronger Teams: When people from various backgrounds come together, they bring unique strengths that complement each other. This creates a more resilient and adaptable team, better equipped to handle the challenges of modern healthcare.

For the last ten years of my tenure, I was fortunate to be a Tier I leader of my direct reports, and this speaks to the importance of a diversified team and our success. As a nurse-COO, I had eleven direct reports, and together, we oversaw 1500+ employees.

Of my eleven directors, 50% were men (nationally 90% of nurses are women), 40% were nurses of color, and 30% identified as LGBTQ+. This diverse team was not just a collection of individuals—it was a powerhouse of talent and perspectives.

- •Gender Balance: Having men in leadership roles brought a different set of skills and experiences to the table. Their strategic thinking, problem-solving, and direct communication styles complemented the strengths of our female leaders, creating a well-rounded leadership team.

- •Cultural and Ethnic Diversity: Our team included nurses of color, who brought invaluable insights into the unique challenges faced by diverse patient populations. This diversity allowed us to develop more culturally sensitive care practices and better serve our community.

- LGBTQ+ Representation: Our LGBTQ+-identifying leaders played a crucial role in fostering an inclusive environment where every employee felt valued and supported. This led to higher morale, lower turnover rates, and a more engaged workforce.

One evening, we faced a sudden influx of patients due to a nearby accident. The emergency room was overwhelmed, and tensions were running high. As the situation escalated, I noticed one of our male directors, John, stepping up. He had a military background and quickly took charge, organizing the response with precision. Meanwhile, our director of cultural competency, Maria, ensured that the needs of our diverse patient population were met with sensitivity and care.

John's strategic approach and Maria's cultural expertise combined to create a seamless response. The team worked tirelessly, and not a single patient was turned away. It was a moment that highlighted the power of diversity in action. Each leader brought something unique to the table, and together, we turned what could have been a chaotic disaster into a coordinated triumph.

Together, this diverse team achieved remarkable success. We consistently met or exceeded our goals, and our patients experienced higher levels of care. The diversity of our leadership was a key factor in our ability to innovate and adapt to the ever-changing healthcare landscape.

One of the most important steps in building a diverse team is the interview process. Ensure your candidates are interviewed by a diverse group of leaders. Candidates will be more comfortable when they can connect with others who have similar experiences, cultural backgrounds, gender, ethnicity, etc.

- **Diverse Interview Panels:** Having a diverse interview panel sends a strong message to candidates about the value your organization places on diversity. It also helps candidates feel more comfortable and confident, knowing they will be working alongside people who share their experiences or backgrounds.

- **Bias Mitigation:** Diverse interview panels can help mitigate unconscious bias. When multiple perspectives are involved in the evaluation process, the likelihood of overlooking qualified candidates based on stereotypes is reduced.

- **Connecting on Common Ground:** Candidates who see themselves represented in the interview panel are more likely to feel a sense of belonging and connection. This can lead to better retention rates and a more engaged workforce.

Looking to the Future: A Brighter Tomorrow for Men in Nursing Leadership

The future of men in nursing leadership is bright, but there's still work to be done. By continuing to advocate for diversity, support aspiring male nurse leaders, and challenge stereotypes, we can create a more inclusive and equitable healthcare system.

- **Ongoing Advocacy:** Advocacy groups and networks play a crucial role in supporting male nurses and leaders. These organizations provide resources, networking opportunities, and professional development, helping to build a robust pipeline of diverse leaders.
- **Inclusive Policies:** Organizations must implement and enforce inclusive policies that ensure fair and equitable treatment for all employees, regardless of gender, race, or sexual orientation. This includes equal access to leadership roles, mentorship programs, and career advancement opportunities.
- **Education and Awareness:** Education and awareness campaigns are essential for challenging stereotypes and promoting nursing as a rewarding career for men. Schools,

healthcare organizations, and media outlets should actively promote the diverse faces of nursing leadership.

- **Celebrating Success:** Finally, we must celebrate the success of male nurse leaders who have broken through barriers and made a difference. I know how often this comes up, but celebration is truly both rewarding and inspirational. Their stories inspire others and help pave the way for future generations.

Embracing diversity in leadership is not just about ticking boxes—it's about creating a stronger, more resilient healthcare system. By fostering a culture of inclusion and supporting diverse leaders, we can ensure that every voice is heard, every perspective is valued, and every patient receives the best possible care.

CHAPTER 14
CREATING A PATHWAY FOR MEN IN LEADERSHIP

The journey to attracting and retaining men in nursing leadership requires a nuanced and multi-pronged approach. It's not enough to simply acknowledge their historical presence; we must actively cultivate their participation and create a welcoming and supportive environment. Think of it not as casting a wider net, but as understanding the ecosystem and using the right lures. Strategic recruitment initiatives are paramount.

We must move beyond traditional methods and forge partnerships with schools, colleges, and veterans' organizations, reaching potential candidates who may never have considered nursing as a viable career path. These collaborations offer a unique opportunity to introduce men to the diverse and rewarding aspects of the profession, dispelling misconceptions and showcasing the potential for growth and leadership. Financial barriers, often a significant hurdle, can be addressed through targeted scholarships and financial aid packages designed specifically for men pursuing nursing degrees. This investment not only makes the profession more accessible but also signals a commitment to supporting their aspirations.

Complementing these initiatives, hands-on experiences, such as shadowing and internships, provide a crucial window into the daily realities of nursing, demystifying the work and allowing potential candidates to envision themselves in the role. Imagine a young man, driven by a desire to help others, discovering a fulfilling career through a simple shadowing experience – that's the transformative power of these opportunities.

But recruitment is just the beginning. We must actively dismantle the outdated stereotypes that continue to plague the profession. Impactful awareness campaigns, leveraging the reach of media and social media platforms, are essential. These campaigns must showcase the diverse and successful male nurse leaders who are already making significant contributions to healthcare. Their stories, amplified through public speaking engagements, conferences, and community events, challenge preconceived notions and normalize the presence of men in nursing.

Picture a national campaign featuring these inspiring figures, sharing their personal journeys, highlighting the unique challenges they've overcome, and demonstrating the profound impact they've had on their patients and the profession. Strategic partnerships with influencers, celebrities, and athletes who champion healthcare can further amplify this message, reaching broader audiences and sparking positive conversations about nursing as a rewarding and respected career choice for men.

Creating a supportive and inclusive environment is paramount for retaining men in nursing and nurturing their leadership potential. Incentives and support systems play a crucial role in this process. Well-defined career advancement programs, complete with mentorship opportunities, specialized training, and access to professional development resources, provide a clear pathway for men to progress beyond bedside care and into leadership positions. This not only benefits individual nurses but also strengthens the profession as a whole by fostering a diverse leadership pipeline. Flexible work schedules and remote work options are also essential, recognizing the diverse responsibilities and commitments that men often juggle.

Imagine a hospital offering part-time leadership roles or allowing nurses to manage administrative tasks remotely, enabling them to balance their professional aspirations with their personal lives. Equally important are robust support networks. These communities offer a safe space for men in nursing to connect with peers, share experiences, offer and receive mentorship, and find a sense of belonging (because, let's face it, sometimes you just need someone who gets it). A mentorship circle, connecting experienced male nurse leaders with aspiring nurses, can provide invaluable guidance, support, and encouragement, empowering them to navigate the challenges and embrace the opportunities that lie ahead.

By weaving together these essential threads – targeted recruitment strategies, impactful awareness campaigns, and robust support systems – we can create a truly inclusive pathway for men in nursing leadership. It's not simply about attracting them to the profession; it's about fostering their growth, empowering their contributions, and ensuring that their diverse perspectives shape the future of healthcare for the better.

Now, while we're not suggesting a 'men-only' nursing club (though that does sound intriguing...), creating targeted support systems is essential. This holistic approach recognizes that true progress requires not only attracting talent but also nurturing it, supporting it, and celebrating its unique contributions.

Guiding The Next Generation

Mentorship programs act as vital lighthouses, guiding aspiring male nurses through the often-uncharted waters of the profession. Structured mentorship, pairing experienced male nurse leaders with those just starting out, offers invaluable support. Mentors share wisdom gleaned from their own journeys, offering advice, insights, and guidance on developing essential leadership skills.

Peer-to-peer mentorship programs create a powerful sense of community, providing a safe space for men to connect, discuss shared challenges, and exchange best practices.

Imagine a group of male nurses meeting regularly, celebrating successes, and offering mutual support – this camaraderie can be incredibly empowering. Mentorship circles, bringing together men with mentors and peers, offer another effective approach, fostering relationships and providing ongoing support, along with a forum for discussing industry trends and professional development. These structured environments create a strong foundation for success.

Advocacy groups serve as powerful champions, fighting for a more equitable and inclusive nursing landscape. Male nurse advocacy networks provide a much-needed voice, addressing the unique challenges men face in the profession. These networks offer resources, networking opportunities, and professional development, fostering a sense of belonging and connection. Policy advocacy is equally crucial.

These groups work to influence policy changes that promote diversity and inclusion, advocating for equal access to leadership roles, fair compensation, and robust anti-discrimination policies. They push for systemic change, ensuring that policies reflect the rich diversity of the nursing workforce. Visibility and recognition are also key. Highlighting the achievements of male nurse leaders through national campaigns, media appearances, and awards ceremonies challenges stereotypes and inspires others to follow in their footsteps, normalizing the idea of men in nursing leadership.

Role models act as beacons, illuminating the path for aspiring male nurses. Promoting male nurses to visible leadership positions shatters stereotypes and demonstrates that nursing is a viable and fulfilling career path for men. Sharing the stories of these leaders through documentaries, social media, and professional publications provides powerful inspiration, showcasing the breadth of opportunities available and the profound impact male nurses have on their communities.

Creating networking opportunities where men can connect with and learn from successful leaders builds a strong community of support and shared purpose. Conferences, summits, and workshops dedicated to male nurse leadership offer a platform for connection, learning, and collaboration, fostering a sense of belonging and shared mission.

By weaving together these three powerful strands – mentorship, advocacy, and role models – we create a robust ecosystem that nurtures and empowers men in nursing. These interconnected initiatives not only provide the tools and resources for success but also foster a strong sense of community and belonging, enabling men to break through barriers, challenge outdated stereotypes, and thrive in leadership roles within this vital and evolving profession.

Building Diversity and Inclusion in Leadership Pipelines

Building a diverse leadership pipeline in nursing requires a multi-pronged approach – it's not a one-size-fits-all situation (unlike those hospital gowns!). Here's the plan:

Early engagement is key. Organizations should nurture the leadership potential of men in nursing from day one. Think leadership training, mentoring (from both men and women – diversity of thought is important!), and real-world opportunities to shine. This shows a career path beyond the bedside, which is crucial for retention. Leadership competency models should be inclusive, valuing diverse leadership styles – emotional intelligence and cultural competence are just as important as technical skills. And don't forget succession planning! Identify promising male nurses early and give them tailored development, so they're ready to lead when the time comes.

Inclusive hiring practices are a must. Blind resume reviews help ditch unconscious bias – qualifications should speak for themselves. Diverse interview panels are also essential, offering different perspectives and making candidates feel more comfortable. Transparency in hiring criteria and processes builds trust and ensures everyone's playing by the same rules.

Regularly assess diversity and inclusion efforts to see what's working and what's not. Be willing to adapt policies and practices – flexibility is key in healthcare (almost as important as hand sanitizer!). Foster a culture of respect, equity, and fairness – it starts at the top. Unconscious bias training can help, and leaders should model inclusive behaviors. Basically, it's about creating a system where everyone has a fair shot at leadership, regardless of gender. Because a diverse leadership team isn't just the right thing to do; it's the smart thing to do.

Let's be clear: diversity in nursing leadership isn't just a good idea; it's a must-have. It's the foundation upon which we build a stronger, more innovative, and more compassionate healthcare future. A diverse leadership team, reflecting the rich tapestry of our communities, brings a wealth of perspectives and experiences that lead to better decisions and enhanced patient care. It's about recognizing the inherent value in every individual and creating an environment where everyone feels empowered to contribute their unique talents. This is how we fuel innovation, build a more inclusive workplace, and ensure that the needs of all – patients and staff – are not just met, but exceeded.

The path forward requires continued effort. Organizations must prioritize developing diverse talent pipelines, actively recruiting and mentoring aspiring male nurse leaders. Advocacy groups play a crucial role in championing policies that promote diversity and inclusion, while visibility and recognition of male nurse leaders inspire others to follow in their footsteps. Education and awareness campaigns are essential for challenging outdated stereotypes and showcasing the rewarding career paths available to men in nursing.

Ultimately, the impact of men in nursing leadership ripples throughout the profession. They serve as role models, break down barriers, and advocate for positive change. Their presence enriches the profession, creating a more welcoming and inclusive environment for future generations of nurses.

As you consider your own role in shaping the future of nursing, ask yourself: How can I contribute to building a more diverse and inclusive leadership pipeline? What actions can I take to support aspiring male nurse leaders and challenge the stereotypes that still persist? Remember, creating a truly equitable and representative healthcare system is a collective responsibility. Every action, no matter how small, contributes to the larger goal of empowering diverse voices and ensuring that everyone has the opportunity to lead and make a difference.

CONCLUSION

"We lose the precious sense that an end is only a beginning in disguise."
–Craig D. Lounsbrough

The end of a thing can be really bittersweet; however, it is quite refreshing to know that the ending of this book could signify the beginning of your journey as a nursing leader. This book has been more than a collection of ideas; it has been an exploration of what it means to be a nursing leader. We've navigated the intricacies of communication, the weight of decision-making, the art of building resilient teams, and the delicate balance of advocacy and patient-centered care. Leadership in nursing isn't just about titles or authority—it's about showing up, standing up, and stepping forward even when the path ahead feels uncertain. If there's one truth that has emerged, it's that leadership is not a fixed destination. It's not a badge you earn and wear forever without effort. It's a living, breathing journey—one that requires continuous learning, unlearning, and relearning. It evolves with each challenge, each patient, each difficult conversation, and every moment that calls on you to be more than you were yesterday.

Take a moment to reflect: What resonated most with you? What insights have shifted your perspective? More importantly, how do you see yourself in this vast and evolving landscape of nursing leadership? Because, make no mistake, you are already a part of it. Whether you realize it or not, your words, your actions, and your presence in healthcare shape the world around you.

Change is a constant in nursing. New policies emerge, technology advances, patient needs evolve, and healthcare itself is in a perpetual state of transformation. In the midst of this, one thing separates great nursing leaders from the rest: their ability to embrace growth. Not as an occasional event, but as a mindset, a way of life. A growth mindset is what allows leaders to turn challenges into opportunities, failures into lessons, and uncertainty into innovation.

Think of a nurse who steps into a leadership role for the first time. They're excited, but self-doubt lurks in the shadows. Maybe they struggle with delegation, or perhaps they freeze when difficult conversations arise. Some might see these as signs they're not cut out for leadership. But a leader with a growth mindset? They see these moments as stepping stones. They reflect, ask questions, seek mentorship, and—most importantly—they push forward. Because they understand that leadership is not about being perfect from the start; it's about evolving every step of the way.

Dr. Carol Dweck, a psychologist known for her work on mindset theory, describes a growth mindset as the belief that abilities and intelligence are not fixed—they can be developed through effort, learning, and persistence. This is particularly true in nursing leadership, where adaptability is as crucial as clinical expertise. No leader, no matter how experienced, has all the answers. The best ones are those who never stop learning, never stop seeking feedback, and never stop striving to improve.

Adopting this mindset isn't always easy. It requires self-awareness. It means recognizing when fear of failure holds you back. It means being willing to say, "I don't know—yet." It means seeking constructive feedback, even when it stings. And most importantly, it means taking action. The best leaders actively challenge themselves. They ask, How can I improve? What lesson can I take from this? How do I turn this setback into growth?

A great way to cultivate a growth mindset is through reflection. Take a moment to think about your leadership journey so far. What challenges have you faced? How have you grown? What lessons have shaped you? Writing these down can be a powerful exercise. In doing so, you start to recognize that every difficulty has been a stepping stone to your current level of expertise. If you've grown before, you can grow again—and again.

Another essential element is mentorship. Surround yourself with people who challenge and inspire you. Seek guidance from those who have walked the path before you. No leader succeeds alone. Learning from others' experiences can provide fresh perspectives and insights that accelerate your growth. At the same time, be open to mentoring others. Teaching what you've learned reinforces your own development and strengthens the entire nursing community.

And let's not forget one of the most important aspects of a growth mindset—resilience. Nursing leadership comes with its fair share of setbacks. Maybe a patient outcome doesn't go as planned, maybe a team conflict arises, or maybe an initiative you spearheaded falls flat. These moments sting, but they are not the end of your journey. They are simply detours. The strongest leaders aren't the ones who never fall—they're the ones who get back up, armed with new knowledge and a deeper sense of purpose.

The beauty of a growth mindset is that it makes leadership sustainable. Burnout is real, and the pressure of leadership can sometimes feel overwhelming. But when you see growth as an ongoing process, you remove the unrealistic expectation that you must have everything figured out today. You allow yourself grace. You recognize that every misstep, every challenge, and every success is simply part of the journey.

As you continue on your leadership path, ask yourself: How can I embrace the ebb and flow of growth? How can I challenge myself to step outside my comfort zone? How can I turn today's struggles into tomorrow's strengths?

The answer lies in adopting the mindset that almost every great leader has embraced: You are not finished. You are always growing. And that, more than anything, is what will set you apart.

With this mindset in place, you're not just preparing for leadership—you're living it. And from here, the next step is clear: putting that growth into action.

The knowledge you've gained isn't meant to sit on a shelf, gathering dust. Leadership is not a theory to be studied in isolation—it's a practice, a way of being. This is where you step forward, take the lessons you've learned, and weave them into the fabric of your daily work. The time for contemplation is over; the time for action is now.

Perhaps this feels daunting. The transition from understanding leadership to embodying it can feel like a steep climb. But here's the good news: leadership doesn't demand grand, theatrical gestures. It starts with small, deliberate choices—choices to be present, to listen, to step up, even when it feels a little uncomfortable. It's in the way you guide a new nurse, advocate for a patient, or navigate a tricky conversation with grace. Every interaction, every decision, every moment is an opportunity to lead.

To guide this transition, set intentional goals. These don't have to be monumental; in fact, the best goals often feel within reach yet stretch you just beyond your comfort zone. Maybe you aim to refine your communication, proactively seeking feedback. Perhaps you commit to learning more about healthcare policy to strengthen your advocacy. Or maybe you decide to mentor a newer nurse, offering guidance and support. These small, consistent steps build a foundation for lasting impact.

A Personal Leadership Development Plan (PLDP) can help structure this process. Think of it as a roadmap—one that keeps you accountable to your growth. What specific skills do you want to develop? What resources will you use? Document your intentions and regularly reassess your progress. This is a living document, evolving with you.

Leadership isn't a solitary endeavor; it thrives in community. Connect with others! Engage with leadership forums, nursing associations, and online communities. The collective wisdom of those who have walked this path can be invaluable. Their insights, encouragement, and even constructive criticism will help you navigate the inevitable challenges.

Equally important is consistency. Leadership isn’t something you switch on and off. True leaders demonstrate integrity and dependability, even when no one is watching. It’s easy to lead when things are smooth sailing, but the real test comes in moments of pressure, conflict, and uncertainty. How you show up then defines your impact.

And let's be real – resilience is key. Nursing leadership will test you. There will be setbacks, resistance, and days that make you question everything (including your choice of career…just kidding…mostly). But resilience isn't about avoiding failure; it's about learning from it. It's about using those missteps as fuel for growth. Some of the most effective leaders faced obstacles, weathered challenges, and chose to rise despite them. Leadership is less about perfection and more about perseverance. So, when you stumble—and you will—dust yourself off and keep going. Let every challenge sharpen you, refine you, and strengthen your resolve.

At this moment, you stand at a crossroads. You can close this book and move on, or you can take what you've learned and breathe life into it. The choice is yours.

So, what's your first step? How will you apply what you've learned? What kind of leader do you want to be? These are not rhetorical questions. They are invitations—an open door to a journey only you can take. It's only fair to encourage you to step through it and take charge.

Charting Your Course

The knowledge you've gained from this book is only as powerful as the action you take with it. Leadership isn't just about learning—it's about doing. This is not just the end of a book; it is the beginning of your journey as a nursing leader. The next steps you take, no matter how small, will shape the kind of leader you become. The transition from theory to practice starts now.

So, where do you begin? Start by reflecting on everything you've absorbed. Identify the concepts that resonated most with you, the insights that sparked a new perspective, and the areas where you still have room to grow. Then, translate these reflections into tangible steps.

Here are some actionable ways to begin:

Create a Personal Leadership Development Plan (PLDP): Outline your leadership goals, whether they are short-term or long-term. What kind of leader do you aspire to be? What qualities do you want to refine? Document your objectives and revisit them regularly to track your progress.

Find a Mentor or Join a Leadership Network: No leader thrives in isolation. Connect with experienced nurse leaders who can offer guidance, support, and invaluable insights. Join professional networks where you can learn from others and share your own experiences.
Set Small, Achievable Leadership Goals: Rome wasn't built in a day, and neither is strong leadership. Start with manageable goals—perhaps taking initiative on a small project, mentoring a junior nurse, or enhancing team communication.

Embrace Accountability and Consistency: Leadership isn't just about grand gestures; it's about showing up every day with the intention to lead by example. Hold yourself accountable for your decisions and actions, even when challenges arise.
Apply What You've Learned: Theory is just the foundation—real growth happens when you implement these lessons in daily practice. Take on leadership roles, spearhead initiatives, advocate for patient care improvements, and cultivate a culture of teamwork and support.

Every challenge is an opportunity to lead.

Final Self-Assessment

Before you embark on your leadership journey, let's take a moment for some honest self-reflection with your pen and journal, of course. I should let you know that this isn't about judging where you are; it's about illuminating where you could be. If it's worth anything, you've gotten this far and it shows you're a go-getter. Think of this as a compass and map, helping you chart your course toward impactful leadership.

Instead of simple yes/no answers, consider how you demonstrate these qualities. Give yourself a rating of 1-5 for each question (1 = Needs significant development, 5 = Consistently demonstrates). And most importantly, jot down specific examples in your journal to illustrate your points. This will make the self-assessment much more valuable.

a) Seeking Feedback: Do I actively solicit feedback from peers, mentors, and team members to refine my leadership skills? (1-5 Rating) How do I do this? What kind of feedback do I seek?
b) Conflict Navigation: How effectively do I handle conflict within my team or workplace? Do I approach it with a

problem-solving mindset? (1-5 Rating) Describe a recent conflict and how you handled it.

c) Embracing Change: Am I open to continuous learning and willing to adapt to the ever-changing landscape of healthcare? (1-5 Rating) How do I stay current with industry trends and adapt my practice accordingly?

d) Leading by Example: Do I embody the values I want to see in my team? (1-5 Rating) What values are most important to me as a leader, and how do I demonstrate them?

e) Responding to Setbacks: How do I respond to setbacks? Do I see them as learning opportunities or as discouraging failures? (1-5 Rating) Describe a time you faced a setback and what you learned from it.

f) Identifying Strengths and Weaknesses: Have I identified my key leadership strengths and areas for development? Am I actively working on improvement? (1-5 Rating) What are my top 3 strengths and 1 area I'm actively working to improve?

g) Advocacy: Do I advocate for my patients, my colleagues, and the profession as a whole? (1-5 Rating) Give an example of a time you advocated for something you believed in.

h) Goal Setting: Have I set clear professional and leadership goals for myself? (1-5 Rating) What are my short-term and long-term leadership goals?

i) Empowering Others: How do I encourage and uplift others around me? Do I create a positive and inclusive work environment? (1-5 Rating) What specific actions do I take to create a positive and inclusive environment?

j) Embracing Challenges: Am I willing to step outside my comfort zone and take on new leadership challenges? (1-5 Rating) What challenges am I currently seeking out or considering taking on?

If you find yourself with lower ratings in some areas, don't worry! This self-assessment is a starting point for charting your course toward becoming the leader you aspire to be. Use your reflections to create a PLDP. Focus on small, achievable steps. Every effort you make, every skill you hone, brings you closer to unlocking your full leadership potential. The journey awaits – are you ready to lead?

Your Next Chapter Begins

After taking the final self-assessment (which, let's be honest, I can't force you to do—you have full autonomy), one truth remains: leadership is not just about personal growth. It's about impact. Every decision you make, every conversation you have, and every challenge you navigate sends ripples through your team, your patients, and the healthcare system as a whole. By fostering collaboration, advocating for better patient care, and mentoring others, you are shaping the future of nursing leadership—whether you realize it or not.

Your leadership journey is uniquely yours. It won't look like anyone else's, nor should it. It will be shaped by your experiences, strengths, and aspirations. There will be wins, setbacks, and moments where you question your path. But great leaders aren't defined by perfection; they're shaped by resilience, self-awareness, and the courage to keep moving forward.

So, take the first step. Then the next. Whether it's seeking mentorship, leading a small initiative, or simply committing to daily self-reflection, every action compounds over time. As John C. Maxwell wisely said,

"The secret of your success is determined by your daily agenda."

And if there's one lesson to carry with you, let it be this:

"Leadership is not about being in charge. It is about taking care of those in your charge." —Simon Sinek

Nursing leadership isn't about titles or power—it's about service. It's about showing up with integrity, clarity, and a commitment to others. It's about being the person people look to in moments of uncertainty, the one who brings steadiness when chaos threatens to take over. Leadership is what happens in the quiet moments between the big decisions—when you advocate for a patient who can't speak for themselves, support a struggling colleague, or ask a hard question that needs to be addressed.

Every shift, every interaction, every challenge is an opportunity to step into your leadership story. Whether you are a new nurse learning to find your voice or a seasoned professional shaping the next generation, your influence matters.

So, you should ask yourself:

What kind of leader do you want to be?

What values will define your leadership?

And more importantly—what one small step can you take today to move closer to that vision?

Because leadership doesn't start in grand moments; it begins in the smallest of choices.

The next chapter of your journey is yours to write. Lead with purpose. Lead with passion. And most importantly—lead with heart.

REFERENCE SECTION:

- Journal Articles:
- "Impact of Nurse Leaders Behaviors on Nursing Staff Performance"
- International Journal of Nursing Sciences, 2023.
- This study explores how nursing leadership behaviors influence nurse performance, emphasizing the critical role of effective leadership in healthcare settings.
- "Engaging Leadership and Nurse Well-being: The Role of the Work Environment"
- Human Resources for Health, 2023.
- This article examines the impact of leadership behavior on nurse well-being, highlighting the importance of supportive work environments.
- "Relationships Between Nursing Leadership and Organizational, Staff, and Patient Outcomes"
- Journal of Nursing Management, 2023.
- A systematic review assessing how different nursing leadership styles are associated with various outcomes in healthcare settings.
- "Impact of Nurse Manager Leadership Styles on Work Engagement"

- Nursing Research and Practice, 2023.
- This review found a significant correlation between positive nurse manager leadership styles and the work engagement of registered nurses.
- "The Impact of Transformational Leadership Style on Nurses' Job Satisfaction"
- SAGE Open Nursing, 2023.
- This review assesses the impact of transformational leadership style on the job satisfaction of hospital nurses.

Books:

- "The Nurse Leader Handbook: The Art and Science of Nurse Leadership"
- By Studer Group, 2009.
- A comprehensive guide covering essential skills and strategies for effective nurse leadership.
- "From Manager to Leader: Strategies for Transforming Health Care"
- By Jo Manion, 2005.
- This book provides insights into transitioning from management to leadership roles within healthcare.
- "Quantum Leadership: Advancing Innovation, Transforming Health Care"

- By Tim Porter-O'Grady and Kathy Malloch, 2014.
- An exploration of innovative leadership practices in the evolving healthcare landscape.

Professional Resources:

- American Nurses Association (ANA) – Leadership Resources
- The ANA offers a variety of resources and articles on nursing leadership, including guides on developing leadership skills and understanding leadership roles.
- Journal of Nursing Management
- A peer-reviewed journal covering advances in nursing management and leadership.

www.ingramcontent.com/pod-product-compliance
Lightning Source LLC
LaVergne TN
LVHW052300200926
848481LV00002B/423
9798218627201